MISOGYNY, PROJECTIVE IDENTIFICATION, AND MENTALIZATION

Misogyny, Projective Identification, and Mentalization looks at how the psychoanalytic concepts of projective identification and mentalization may explain the construction of society and how they have enabled misogyny to be expressed in social, political, and institutional settings. Karyne E. Messina explores how misogyny has affected the perception and treatment of women through analysis of a range of examples of individual women and groups.

The first part explores projective identification as a mechanism for the suppression of women, looking at the origins of the concept in psychoanalysis and its expansion. The author examines the story of Clara Thompson as an example, arguing that her virtual disappearance from the history of psychiatry and psychoanalysis itself is a telling example of this process at work. The second part of the book uses four examples of individuals, including the recent election loss by Hillary Clinton in 2016, to show that projective identification can (particularly in political and cultural settings) overtake and motivate groups as well as individuals, and lead to violence, atrocity, humiliation, and dismissal of and against women. Part three then features case studies of four groups of women from the 20th century, including victims of the 1994 Rwandan genocide, showing how projective identification against groups has occurred.

With specific reference to the erasure of women's contributions in society, both individually and collectively, and the trauma that arises from the many effects of regarding women as a group as "less" or "other," this is a book which sets a new agenda for understanding how misogyny is expressed socially. *Misogyny, Projective Identification, and Mentalization* will be of interest to psychoanalysts and psychoanalytic psychotherapists as well as scholars of politics, gender, and cultural studies.

Karyne E. Messina, Ed.D., FABP, is a psychologist and supervising analyst at the Washington Baltimore Center for Psychoanalysis and is on the medical staff of Johns Hopkins Medicine in Bethesda, Maryland, USA. She maintains a full-time private practice in Chevy Chase, Maryland. She was previously the Director of the Meyer Treatment Center at the Washington School of Psychiatry and the Director of Continuing Education for Women at George Washington University.

"This book presents novel ideas that advance not only the understanding of projective identification, but also concepts related to the aspects of work that promote improvement in psychotherapy that I have not seen before. I think that the topics of the book will be of universal interest to a variety of readers for many years to come, as the issue of discrimination not only continues to be a struggle, but in recent times, the 'Me Too' movement gives these questions urgency not seen before. The book contains a very contemporary application of theory on social experience; it is likely to become a tour de force work."
  Harry Gill, Assistant Clinical Professor, George Washington University; Medical Director, Suburban Hospital, Johns Hopkins Medicine, USA

"Here Karyne E. Messina explores misogyny through a psychoanalytic lens. Familiar with many theoretical perspectives and using wide-ranging examples, she shows how psychoanalytic theories contribute to an understanding of misogyny's unconscious roots and its potential for resolution. The reader is guaranteed a thoughtful, thorough and suspenseful journey through this timely topic."
  Helen Stein (retired), Consultant, New York State Psychiatric Institute, Center for the Study of Trauma and Resilience; Psychologist, private practice, New York City, USA

"In this important book, psychoanalyst Karyne E. Messina describes the damaging effects of what she calls the 'emotional violence of silence', the deployment of power to erase the contribution of women throughout history. Today in the age of the 'Me Too' movement, women are starting to speak out—but the rising tide of voices still has to combat a long history of systemic suppression. Understanding these forces has never been more timely. This book can help us break the cycle and usher in a new and necessary cultural shift."
  Maddie Grant, Culture Consultant and Digital Strategist and Founding Partner, WorkXO, Washington, DC, USA

"Dr. Messina's book takes up the worryingly persistent problem of misogyny. Marshaling several rich examples, she shows how the process of projective identification illuminates diverse manifestations of violence against women. Drawing on attachment theory, she explains how self-awareness and perspective-taking can allow us to escape the grips of projective identification and potentially ameliorate the continuing prejudicial ways women are treated. This book makes an important contribution to further our understanding of the problem of misogyny."
  Shweta Sharma, Assistant Professor in the Menninger Department of Psychiatry & Behavioral Sciences at Baylor College of Medicine; Staff Psychologist at the Menninger Clinic, Houston, Texas, USA

MISOGYNY, PROJECTIVE IDENTIFICATION, AND MENTALIZATION

Psychoanalytic, Social, and Institutional Manifestations

Karyne E. Messina

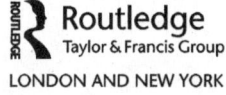

LONDON AND NEW YORK

First published 2019
by Routledge
2 Park Square, Milton Park, Abingdon, Oxon, OX14 4RN

and by Routledge
52 Vanderbilt Avenue, New York, NY 10017

Routledge is an imprint of the Taylor & Francis Group, an informa business

© 2019 Karyne E. Messina

The right of Karyne E. Messina to be identified as author of this work has been asserted by her in accordance with sections 77 and 78 of the Copyright, Designs and Patents Act 1988.

All rights reserved. No part of this book may be reprinted or reproduced or utilised in any form or by any electronic, mechanical, or other means, now known or hereafter invented, including photocopying and recording, or in any information storage or retrieval system, without permission in writing from the publishers.

Trademark notice: Product or corporate names may be trademarks or registered trademarks, and are used only for identification and explanation without intent to infringe.

British Library Cataloguing-in-Publication Data
A catalogue record for this book is available from the British Library

Library of Congress Cataloging-in-Publication Data
Names: Messina, Karyne E., author.
Title: Misogyny, projective identification, and mentalization : psychoanalytic, social, and institutional manifestations / Karyne E. Messina.
Description: Abingdon, Oxon ; New York, NY : Routledge, 2019. | Includes bibliographical references and index.
Identifiers: LCCN 2018056882 (print) | LCCN 2018058825 (ebook) | ISBN 9780367192235 (e-Book) | ISBN 9780429578793 (Adobe) | ISBN 9780429574573 (Mobipocket) | ISBN 9780429576683 (ePub) | ISBN 9780367192143 (hardback : alk. paper) | ISBN 9780367192211 (pbk. : alk. paper)
Subjects: LCSH: Projective identification. | Misogyny. | Metacognition.
Classification: LCC RC455.4.P76 (ebook) | LCC RC455.4.P76 M47 2019 (print) | DDC 616.89–dc23
LC record available at https://lccn.loc.gov/2018056882

ISBN: 978-0-367-19214-3 (hbk)
ISBN: 978-0-367-19221-1 (pbk)
ISBN: 978-0-367-19223-5 (ebk)

Typeset in Bembo
by Swales & Willis, Exeter, Devon, UK

CONTENTS

Prologue: the dig   *viii*
Preface   *x*
Acknowledgments   *xii*

Introduction: beginnings   1

PART I
One mechanism that explains our violent world   9

1 A mechanism that harms: projective identification as a force that destroys   11

2 Clara Thompson's disappearance: how projective identification contributed to the near-extinction of a star   21

PART II
Those who have been damaged: projective identification as a major cause of the erasure   43

3 Eleanor Marx: a little-known activist   45

4 A 21st century woman: Anne Case   53

5 Hillary Clinton and the 2016 presidential election   64

PART III
Groups of women who have been damaged: the effects of projective identification in groups   **77**

6 The dial painters and their fate: illness and death for many   79

7 The WASP of World War II: does the stigma linger?   87

8 The challenge: healing groups and cultures   94

9 The atrocities of physical abuse: genocide and rape in Rwanda and sex-trafficked girls   99

PART IV
Mechanisms that reverse the damage: mentalization and reparative leadership as antidotes to projective identification   **109**

10 Attachment, attachment trauma, and mentalization: key components that affect the development of the self and the formation of group identity   111

11 Reparative leadership as a way to help groups: reconciliation in Rwanda as an example of hope   122

PART V
Attempting to turn things around: from projective identification (a one-mind process) to mentalization (a two-minds process)   **129**

12 Treatment out of the analytic box: attachment, mentalization, and a response to trauma   131

13 The lady—as my observing ego—and I: observing mentalization after forming attachment relationships   137

Conclusion   153

Epilogue: a new collaboration   162

Index   165

PROLOGUE
The dig

As if I were an underwater archeologist, I've been on a lot of diving "digs." Often as a young child I went to sites to be explored by boat. I became increasingly curious about the flora and exotically colored fish to be found there, as well as the jagged rocks that hurt my feet. The unique coral formations fascinated me, I think because I learned early that these spiky, piercing, once-living peaks of coral rock were forged together, creating the foundation on which the Florida Keys were built.

In my experience as a child, what mattered most, beyond the safety provided by my parents, was the fascinating natural environment with its tropical breezes, palm trees, and wondrous objects to study. I was curious too about the people who made their way to my island in the sun. Some, it seemed, came from afar to reinvent themselves, others simply sought the peace and quiet of a tropical paradise. There was something intriguing about contact with these people, in the context of exploring my universe, that was filled with possibility. I came to realize for the first time that who I was as a person was based on everything I had experienced in life up to that very moment in time. And it was in the Keys that I first came to know that people are the way they are because of what life has brought to them, starting with their original environment.

As an adult my focus shifted to ideas and concepts of the mind. At that point the "digs" usually were related to aspects of psychology, psychoanalysis, philosophy, and other areas of study that explain "what makes us tick" as inhabitants of the earth. Frequently, when I've wandered a bit from familiar territory, these detours have led me to beautifully creative works of wonder, such as activists' brave efforts for social justice as agents of change, and an amazing host of ideas and theories that became fascinating new aspects of my internal world.

Wherever my curiosity has taken me, I have found that much of what has been discovered, conceptualized, invented, designed, accomplished, or composed was the work—so say the reports and histories—of men. No great numbers of women have been found on my mental "digs." But how could that be? I've often wondered.

Throughout history in many fields of study, women have mysteriously disappeared from memory despite the contributions they have made. At times and in some fields, women seem hardly to have existed at all. I've been increasingly puzzled by this phenomenon: How could it be possible that only men have been ever-present as heroes, inventors, discoverers, great scientists, and philosophers? More and more often in my own field of psychoanalytic therapy, this disappearance has been brought home to me. Women historians in many fields have, of course, asked the same question. They've found powerful answers, but the issue persists.

For centuries women have weathered storms of underestimation, disrespect, and character assassination, usually at the hands of men. Even after the advent of second-wave feminism, critics have undermined the contributions of women to society and culture. When women suggest an idea, propose change, or develop something that challenges the status quo (especially if the unfamiliar idea shows promise), the men who benefit from existing habits and systems often resist. When women's ideas disappear, violence has been done to their minds and spirits, in psychic blows that cannot heal as the body does. While it goes without saying that there have been some positive changes that have occurred over the years, people like Gloria Steinem have indicated that progress does not occur as fast as one might suspect (Hass, 2011).

The news as well continually presents me with outrageous, inexplicable findings. No one cause can explain sexual trafficking of young women, dismissal of women pilots who served the American military, or casual corporate denial of the health concerns of working-class women. The same is true, in a painfully personal, usually secretive form, for individual women whose reputations and even lives are silenced by ideological and professional competitors, by lovers, by any man of ill will whom they unconsciously threaten—and their plight is rarely in the news.

I have developed my own melancholy image: Women have been part of life's voyage throughout the centuries, but on the vessel's manifest, their names are frequently no longer visible. If ever they were there in the first place, they have been worn away. It is as if the little boat that took me to my islands of wonder as a child had initials carved on its gunwales, but only those of the boys have endured; the etchings of the girls faded long ago. This book explores one of the processes by which this erasure came about.

PREFACE

My curiosity about this topic began when I was the director of the Meyer Treatment Center at the Washington School of Psychiatry several years ago. While writing a commentary for the journal *Psychiatry* (Spring 2014), I became interested in Clara Thompson, one of the School's founders, who seemed to get little credit for her many contributions. Thereafter I developed an interest in researching the lives of other women (and groups of women) who have not received recognition for their work. A theory about this "erasure" and hypotheses as to how this process could be changed are also included in my thinking.

While President Trump appears in various parts of this book, it is not about him *per se*; it is broader than the life or influence of any one person. Where his name does appear, it is there to illustrate a dynamic that has been part of the human story for ages.

Ultimately, this book is about the power some have over others. In most cases the stories I tell concern women, because historically women have occupied a subordinate position. It is my hope that my readers will be able to use the concepts described in this book to identify the individual struggles they have had with another person or other people. If one can better understand the negative mechanisms that are involved in any relationship, I believe, communication can improve and tensions can be reduced.

When engaged in a process of understanding others, people do not have to agree. What is essential, if we are to improve connections between and among ourselves, is mutual respect, untainted by judgment. We must allow people, regardless of age, gender, or race, to have opinions of their own. Agreement is much more likely to be achieved when we know ourselves, accept the differences that exist among and between us, and together try to establish a third idea that incorporates aspects of both perspectives. It is, after all, through mutual agreement that buy-in emerges.

The concept of "violence" in my book is used to illustrate how various types of acts against others fit into this category, e.g., how acts of dismissal can threaten one's inner sense of being in much the same way as physical actions can endanger one's entire self, external and internal. As an age-old phenomenon it is ubiquitous and incessant as well as protean, varying its outward form according to the social constellation at hand. In *Topology of Violence*, the philosopher Byung-Chul Han (2018) considers the shift in violence from the visible to the invisible, from the frontal to the viral to the self-inflicted, from brute force to mediated force, from the real to the virtual. Anonymized, desubjectified, systemic violence conceals itself because it has become embedded in society.

Violence, Han (2018) tells us, has gone from the negative—explosive, massive, and martial—to the positive, wielded without enmity or domination. This, he says, creates the false impression that violence has disappeared. Han (2018) investigates the macro-physical manifestations of violence, developing from the tension between self and other, interior and exterior, friend and enemy. It runs the gamut, he explains, from merciless torture to the bloodless violence of the gas chamber, the faceless brutality of terrorism, and the psychic blows of hurtful language.

ACKNOWLEDGMENTS

I would like to extend my gratitude to the people who made this book possible. They include Dr. Alec Whyte, who introduced me to the Washington School of Psychiatry many years, Dr. Harry Gill, former Executive Director of the Washington School, and Paul Gill, who supported my effort to undertake and complete this project. I also want to acknowledge Dr. Ann-Louise Silver, who read many early versions of the chapter on Clara Thompson, a nearly forgotten early Director of the School. I am also grateful to Dr. Jon Allen, who generously provided guidance whenever I needed expert advice about attachment theory and mentalization, and to Dr. Abbie O. Smith, my mentor and friend, who has devoted her life to championing the rights of women. She has been an inspiration to leagues of women.

I am grateful to Routledge staff for their publishing advice, especially Kate Hawes and Charles Bath, who enthusiastically supported this topic. I also greatly appreciate the advice I received from Dr. Michael O'Loughlin, and I also want to thank Dr. Linda Salamon, who spent many hours editing my original manuscript and researching various topics in the book. I am exceedingly grateful to John Knecht, who painstakingly edited my manuscript and provided invaluable advice.

I also want to thank Dr. Marianne Vardalos, for generously giving me permission to reprint excerpts from my chapter, *The Despair and Hope in Projective Identification*, which originally was published in 2009 in *Engaging terror: A critical and interdisciplinary approach*.

Last by not least I want to thank my family for their help and support: my husband, Gary, for his excellent editorial advice and my lawyer daughters. Kiki Messina, who as a prosecutor in a special victims unit, helped contribute to my understanding of human trafficking, domestic violence, and child abuse and Ann-Kathryn So, who provided invaluable information about various aspects of discrimination against women. I also want to thank Isabel, Olivia, and Christopher, who will make great contributions to the world someday. They inspire me every day.

INTRODUCTION

Beginnings

In order to do one's job effectively and reflectively, whether as a psychologist, neuroscientist, artist, or king, one needs a philosophy and theory of mind. How is knowledge gathered, tested, absorbed by the conscious mind? I explore not only cognitive knowledge but emotional, "executive," and even physical knowledge.

As a psychoanalyst I believe we are the sum total of what we have experienced: through the senses, through encounters with other people beginning with our parents, through reading and the arts, through team or individual sports, for some through a spiritual life. As individuals navigating in a world filled with unimaginable radiance on one end of the continuum and incomprehensible pain on the other, we can only know what we have experienced, firsthand or through observation. The subjective experience reigns. Yet it is important to keep in mind that it is in conjunction with another (or others) that we come to know who we are, what we know, and what we feel. It is a complex web of knowing that has been bestowed on us by our genetic heritage.

At the same time, knowledge is inevitably cultural: we can only experience what the society around us offers. We also need a level of what Fonagy, Luyten and Campbell (2014) call "epistemic trust," which mean a person's capacity to take in and believe what someone else has said or communicated to him or her without skeptically questioning everything that is said. This capacity, which requires a secure attachment early in life, permits the child to learn cues from his or her environment, i.e., social and cultural cues learned from adults who can mentalize. Thus, the mind escapes solipsism, and its possessor can participate in the culture. Simply put, what it comes down to is trust. In addition to needing to take in information from others to learn about ourselves and our world, we have to trust the source of the information. When we don't, learning is stifled.

Of course, our experiences lead to different kinds of knowing that emerge in our minds; one important element in "knowing" is how we come to learn, subjectively, the content of our minds. Classic psychoanalytic theory suggests that we remember in our conscious minds the good, pleasant aspects of life, whereas many of the unpleasant, painful parts of our experiences reside in our unconscious minds, out of our awareness. Those that are too painful to bear we repress. As a result, some of our actions are triggered by unpleasant memories that reside in unconscious thought. We also cannot know what is unconscious because it is not at our disposal without extensive effort that one expends through free association in psychoanalysis, to name one way in which the unconscious mind becomes conscious.

A significant part of our experience is absorbed from the culture in which we are raised, with all its stereotypes, biases, and prejudices. These aspects of our knowing come in part from what our parents tell us, what we learn at school, from what the media puts before us and from other various types of projections we receive from other people (Messina, 2009). Consider, for example, a recent situation in which highly educated reporters commented on the work of Anne Case and Angus Deaton, well-known economists from Princeton University. These writers assumed that Professor Case was a secondary figure when they described her not as his colleague who had done some of the initial work, but instead as the professor's wife. Dr. Deaton, on the other hand, was mentioned as a winner of the Nobel Prize even though much of his research had been done with Professor Case, who had independently investigated many of the hypotheses that laid the groundwork in the area.

Whatever the case may be, the comments, in my view, were based on events in the reporters' own personal lives or on lifelong exposure to certain notions with respect to the meaning of the word "wife." After all, through centuries of patriarchy, men were automatically thought to be superior. The reporters might have meant precisely what they said because their reactions came from the unconscious part of their minds, where the inequality of genders may be deeply embedded. Some might not even recognize the bias that comes out of their mouths, issues from their keyboards, bias generated by their speech or writing, bias instilled, at least in part, by the words or actions of others.

In a society where prejudice—against women or any racial, religious, or other marginalized group—is tolerated or even promoted, the individual may not consciously recognize the concept of stereotype or bias. The prejudice may not represent how we consciously wish to be in the world but rather what we have gleaned from others. Our attitudes may have congealed in our minds as early as childhood. Such internalizations, whether conscious or unconscious, allow all kinds of violence to be perpetrated against women and others considered inferior. *Associated* thoughts and feelings emanating from prejudice can be projected onto others as well.

In this manuscript I explain the psychoanalytic concepts that contribute to my philosophy of change, forward movement, and cure by analyzing what has happened to the women, and groups of women, whose stories I tell. Their emotions, their character, their very psyches have borne the brunt of psychological violence. Indeed, they themselves in some cases have been the victims of physical violence. In my examples, much of the damage that was done was initiated by men and groups of men. Why, in addition to the cultural prejudices I mentioned earlier, did those men encounter women in the ways that they did? What was it about their own experiences that led them to act viciously, or simply dismissively? I provide explanations of the processes involved as well as illustrations of these psychoanalytic processes as they emerge in everyday life, including projective identification.

I also propose a mindset about working with people that is in accordance with Jon Allen's less-structured way of doing therapy with survivors of trauma (Allen, 2012). It is similar to the way Fonagy and Allen describe mentalizing in *The American Psychiatric Publishing Textbook of Psychiatry* (2014) as well.

While Allen and Fonagy (2006, 2008) have distinguished between mentalizing as a modality of treatment and as a way of interacting with patients that can be useful to therapists regardless of previous theoretical orientation, the inclusion of the definition in a mainstream psychiatric publication appears to be a major step forward for the mental health field. What they have determined, based on research findings accrued over many years, is the fact that patients improve because of the *relationship* they have had with their therapist, regardless of the type of psychotherapy practiced by the treating professional. Hence, Fonagy and Allen (2014) believe all therapists benefit from being able to mentalize with their patients irrespective of technical approach. The capacity to repair ruptures in the therapeutic alliance was another outcome that was found to be significant among all treatment modalities.

> Decades of psychotherapy research have shown a consistent finding; compared with control conditions, many brands of psychotherapy are demonstrably effective, but it is difficult to show consistently that any particular brand is more effective than any other ... Whereas differences among brands generally carry limited weight, extensive evidence attests to the substantial impact of the quality of the patient-therapist relationship on outcomes (Norcross, 2011). Most notably, evidence consistently attests to the importance of the therapeutic alliance. The therapist relationship is what seems to matter (Horvath, Del Re, Flückiger & Symonds, 2011) as well as the capacity to repair ruptures in the alliance (Safran, Muran & Eubanks-Carter, 2010). Our approach is entirely consistent with this emphasis on the therapeutic relationship for which we use the language of mentalizing in the context of a secure attachment relationship.
>
> *(Fonagy & Allen, 2014, p. 1110)*

The expanded way of thinking about mentalizing suggests that a therapist trained in any modality, whether it be psychoanalysis, cognitive or behavioral therapy, or any other (standard) type of treatment can help another person by understanding the patient's problem from his or her vantage point; it's not how the therapist views the issue but how the patient experiences it. This is mentalizing (Fonagy & Allen, 2014).

The work I do with traumatized patients I have called "Treatment Out of the Analytic Box." Jon Allen (2012) has referred to his method as "Plain Old Therapy." Simply put, in both cases there is an emphasis on providing a secure base as well as creating an atmosphere that promotes mentalizing—being aware of one's internal as well as external world while accepting without judgment that others have different views and experiences.

With regard to my own work, I believe that by providing a secure, nonjudgmental environment, as well as by creating an atmosphere in which subjective experiences are valued, I allow my patients to slowly begin to recount their stories. Learning that it is possible for another person to understand their experiences, both internal and external, without judging them is often something new for patients, especially when they come to know that their therapist's experiences are different. In time the new learning I am describing leads to the development of a new capacity, a valuable new skill that helps them understand the mind of another person. This is no small feat for someone who has been abused throughout life in one way or another, which is most often what has occurred when someone has been traumatized.

I will also briefly discuss the renewed relationship between old partners, psychoanalysis and neuroscience (Damasio, 2015), with added information on attachment circuitry (Cozolino, 2006) and the theory of listening (Spunt, 2013).

Description of the book

Throughout my book I illustrate what has happened to many women who have made major contributions to society only to be forgotten. This phenomenon is part of a debate, spanning more than a century, between scholars, psychoanalysts, feminists, and philosophers on the position of women in society. In many fields the work of women has mysteriously disappeared from historical memory. At times and in certain disciplines such as physics and math, women have not had the same opportunities as men. Seldom have they held top positions. With regard to some careers, in the music industry for instance, they seem hardly to have existed at all. There are so few females in audio recording associations that the number of members who are women has not been recorded in the last 15 years (Boboltz, 2016).

But that is very old news; the psychological suffering that results from the emotional violence of silence is evergreen. In my professional observation, deepened by my research, women have weathered storms of underestimation, disrespect, moral degradation, and character assassination, usually at the hands of men. Even after the advent of second-wave feminism, critics—often, though not exclusively, male—have undermined the contributions of women to civil society and culture. I have written this book to gain, and to share, a better understanding of how and why these travesties have occurred.

I begin in Part I by describing projective identification. This mechanism that allows a person or group to get rid of negative feelings, thoughts, or fantasies by attributing them to someone else or to another group. Of course, all such complex events are multidetermined, but unconscious motivation is a powerful explanatory element. The major motivation involved is the psychological need of a person to do away with what cannot be accepted by that person about himself or herself. At work here is the person's psychological need to banish unacceptable aspects of him- or herself, aspects that dwell in that person's unconscious mind. In this case, the failure to accept part of oneself is painful because the unacceptable is perceived as bad. I also describe the life of Clara Thompson in this section for the purpose of illustrating the mechanisms that are at play in projective identification.

In Part II of the manuscript I describe the experiences of individual high-achieving women who have known the type of erasure of which I speak. The era in question dates from 1850 to today and the women include, in addition to Thompson, Eleanor Marx, Hillary Clinton, and Anne Case. I chose women who, with a strong sense of personal agency, threw themselves into events with less reserve than more vulnerable people might have done. They survived, made changes to our world, and accomplished some of their goals along the way. But they also have been marginalized. Thompson, from my own field of psychoanalysis and psychodynamic therapy, was the source of my original question. She contributed a great deal to schools of thought that are associated with current theories subscribed to by relationalists, self-psychologists, interpersonalists, or others who place emphasis on the ideas inherent in mentalizing. However, many scholars as well as therapists in the field have never heard her name. Despite the power and intellect of all four women, Clinton is likely to be the only name recognized by many readers. We cannot yet know the full scope of her accomplishments or those of Case—or how long the memory of them will last.

In Part III I present the tragic experiences and the erasure of four groups of anonymous women over the last century: World War II women pilots (WASP), sex-trafficked girls, female assembly-line workers in radium factories, and Rwandan women who were victims of wartime violence during the genocide of 1994. These groups demonstrate how women in various sociopolitical-cultural settings have suffered physical and emotional damage that has been readily extinguished from the memories of their superiors, handlers, or perpetrators.

The dynamics I describe illustrate how negative, unacceptable thoughts and ideas can be disavowed because they are too painful to bear. With respect to radium, for instance, factory owners were not able to tolerate being responsible for the horrible deaths that befell their female workers. That a dentist could remove a woman's jaw simply by pulling it out with his hand is unthinkable. Some of the same women who worked with radium suffered from shortened legs that then fractured as a result of working with the toxic substance (Moore, 2017).

In the case of human trafficking, I want to raise awareness of atrocities that continue to occur on a daily basis, usually under the radar of most people in the world as well as the media. In the chapters on Rwanda I describe aspects of mentalization: those that prevent and those that facilitate individual thinking by all without judgment. All of these examples should help the reader understand the nature of the complex phenomenon I am addressing.

In Part IV of the book I describe in detail how the concept of projective identification can be related to key ideas associated with attachment and attachment trauma. I also describe how some of the ideas inherent in mentalization, e.g., attachment theory and the theory of listening, if incorporated into the concept of therapeutic action or a theory of cure, can lead to the "taking back of projections." Understanding the mechanisms at play in unconscious and conscious minds can be the first step toward healing from trauma. The recovery of one's capacity to mentalize is a highly useful tool in the treatment of those who have been damaged by projective identification.

In Part V, the final section of the book, I present ways in which the damage of projection can be reversed through the abovementioned process of the taking back of projections. The key to this process, in addition to the acquisition of the capacity to mentalize as discussed in Part I, is the relevance of attachment and the effects of attachment trauma. The need for repair is also discussed. In this section I also present ideas and practices—my own and those of others from whom I have learned so much—about treatment for women and children who have been damaged by or have suffered through the aftermath of emotional or physical violence. This part includes clinical vignettes that demonstrate clearly how my ideas come into play in the treatment of such patients.

For victims, expelling unwanted projections and coming to know what belongs to them and what belongs to the other is essential. These techniques allow people to feel whole again. For perpetrators, vicious internal storms and unwarranted attacks on the other can be halted through mentalizing. When empathizing with others becomes part of the story, changes can occur for individuals and people in groups as well. Extending one's imagination into another's humanity without hesitation or reservation can subdue the inner storm. In the end I describe wrongdoing and underscore the cost to those who have been damaged while postulating a theory of cause and the possibility of hope. I also suggest that the forms of therapy I promote are optimal techniques for some people who have been traumatized, rather than simply promoting the "evidence-based" forms of treatment in current use.

Interspersed throughout the manuscript are also brief connective elements of memoir. Along the way I tell stories from my own life that illustrate the psychoanalytic principles I describe, such as the nature of strong attachment, the threat of mysterious illness, a psychodynamic epistemology, and the effectiveness of women's solidarity when under threat. Although much of what I describe involves the pain and suffering women have endured at the hands of men, I have little doubt that in contemporary circumstances, women can and will behave as illustrated in Margaret Atwood's *The Handmaid's Tale*. This story, which was recently adapted for TV, was initially told in a book written in 1985. It is being revisited because, strangely enough, in this era of Trump, the control of women is appearing to many to reflect future possibilities—where we have been and where we could go again. Hence, it is not just men who have power over women. Women in the middle stratum of various settings can terrorize those beneath them. Atwood herself is distressed by this phenomenon.

To emphasize this point, last year she wrote an article in *The New York Times* (Atwood, 2017) that focused on how women "gang up" on each other to save themselves. She pointed out that this occurs on social media through "swarming," which is when an entire group of people gang up on a single person. A devastating example that comes to my mind is when a group of girls attack another, for example, on Instagram. The results can be devastating and have at times led to suicide due to the feelings of hopelessness that befalls the victim of the social media "attack."

Atwood also wrote about the "aunts" in the story and described them as the sadists, yet also as the true believers who thought they were protecting the Handmaidens from the atrocities of the real world, a mindset that unfortunately is imaginable in today's world.

Recently LGBTQ theorists and scholars in gender studies have criticized the strong binary of male-female that pervades history and culture. I support the efforts of gay, lesbian, and transgender people to destabilize that iron duality. As a feminist I also recognize that, since the 1970s, in psychology "masculine" and "feminine" have been shown by researchers to be the ends of a continuum.

A new term, "redactional identification" is also introduced and defined in Chapter 13. It involves intention and is a way one creates an aspect of himself or herself that is ego-syntonic—a desirable, active and knowable part of the self.

References

Allen, J. G. (2012). *Restoring mentalizing in attachment relationships: Treating trauma with plain old therapy*. Washington, DC: American Psychiatric Association Publishers.

Allen, J. G. & Fonagy, P. (2006). Preface. In J. G. Allen & P. Fonagy (Eds.), *Handbook of mentalization-based treatment* (p. viiiix). New York, NY: John Wiley & Sons.

Allen, J. G., Fonagy, P. & Bateman, A. W. (2008). *Mentalizing in clinical practice*. Washington, DC: American Psychiatric Association Publishing.

Atwood, M. (2017). Margaret Atwood on what *The Handmaid's Tale* means in the age of Trump. *The New York Times*, 10.

Boboltz, S. (2016, May 3). There are so few women in music production, no one bothers to count. *Huffington Post*.

Cozolino, L. (2006). *The neuroscience of human relationships: Attachment and the developing social brain*. New York, NY: Norton.

Damasio, A. (2015, January 12). Neuropsychoanalysis. *Lookup-id.com*. Retrieved from https://lookup-id.com/dir/neuropsychoanalysis.html.

Fonagy, P. & Allen, J. G. (2014). *The American Psychiatric Publishing textbook of psychiatry* (6th ed.). R. Hales, S. Yudofsky & L. Roberts (Eds.). Arlington, VA: American Psychiatric Publishing.

Fonagy, P., Luyten, P., & Campbell, C. (2014, December). Epistemic trust, psychopathology, and the great psychotherapy debate. *Society for the Advancement of Psychotherapy*. Society for Psychotherapy.

Horvath, A. O., Del Re, A. C., Flückiger, C. & Symonds, D. (2011). Alliance in individual psychotherapy. *Psychotherapy, 48*(1), 9.

Messina, K. (2009). Taking back projections: The despair and hope in projective identification. Paper presented at 2nd Annual International Conference on the Human Condition, Barrie, Ontario, May 2008. Published in M. Vardalos (Ed.), *Engaging terror: A critical and interdisciplinary approach*. Boca Raton, FL: Universal Publishers.

Moore, K. (2017). *Radium girls: The dark story of America's shining women*. Naperville, IL: Sourcebooks.

Norcross, J. C. (Ed.). (2011). *Psychotherapy relationships that work: Evidence-based responsiveness* (2nd ed.). New York, NY: Oxford University Press.

Safran, J. D., Muran, J. C. & Eubanks-Carter, C. (2010). Repairing alliance ruptures. In J. C. Norcross (Ed.), *Psychotherapy relationships that work: Evidence-based responsiveness* (2nd ed.) (pp. 224–238). New York, NY: Oxford University Press.

Spunt, R. P. (2013). Mirroring, mentalizing, and the social neuroscience of listening. In *International Journal of Listening 27*(2), 61–72.

PART I
One mechanism that explains our violent world

PART I

1
A MECHANISM THAT HARMS
Projective identification as a force that destroys

Early developments; formation of the idea

Women have accomplished so much, yet our voices are not always heard. When we do manage to rise to the top, we are often silenced. Why does this happen? Do we allow this phenomenon to occur, do we encourage it or is it foisted upon us? My major hypothesis suggests that there is a psychological mechanism at play that causes us to stop short of the finish line or slow down toward the end of the race, primarily because of unconscious forces that push against our forward movement.

At times women are behind the wish to undo the accomplishments of other women, but most often it is men, because of their historical position of power. They perpetuate this process of elimination because of an unfamiliar and unwanted sense of badness, one that they must thrust onto another to preserve themselves.

That said, neither men nor women are inherently bad, but inherent in all of us are aggressive impulses and tendencies that are fraught with explosive possibilities. We can destroy our children, families, and countries, not because we are evil, but rather because we have not modulated, or had modulated for us, aspects of ourselves that are unknowable, aspects we cannot bear. Hence, we project these things outwardly, ridding ourselves of unwanted feelings and ways of being that we do not or cannot accept: the "not-me" parts of ourselves. We see this phenomenon occurring on the current world stage, where all types of actions that are hard to comprehend are directed toward others, from vindictive verbal attacks to horrendous acts of terror. How and why do these things occur? Why are such happenings so ubiquitous? Do we not know what we do to others? How does simple conflict escalate into attempts to annihilate individuals, groups of people, and entire countries?

In an attempt to better understand how these things happen, I will examine this key psychoanalytic concept that is so relevant when trying to make sense of what we see in our world today. Ideas developed by Melanie Klein (1946) can help explain the tendency to disavow and then attribute to others what we cannot tolerate within. The major mechanism that destroys the other is called projective identification. It is primarily a primitive process, one wherein an unacceptable or even monstrous aspect of an individual's internal world must be expelled.

While Klein did not coin the term herself, since it was used earlier by Edoardo Weiss to describe choice of sexual partners (Spillius, 2007), the specific process to which I am referring was described by Klein in 1946 as she was developing her ideas about intrapsychic states of mind she called "positions." Simply put, she was talking about ways in which people experience and relate to each other. In what she called the "paranoid-schizoid" position, Klein (1946) talked about the need to mentally "get rid of" bad, threatening aspects of the self that are too much to bear. From this perspective, others are not experienced as complete or whole with good and bad qualities, but rather as fragmented, i.e., the entirety of that person's being is not acknowledged. In this state, one's own unbearable feelings and thoughts are projected outwardly and thereafter attributed to the other because they cannot be tolerated. In the paranoid-schizoid position, wherein anxiety is intense and mostly persecutory, people figuratively or literally retaliate, seek revenge, hurt, or otherwise "get back at" a person or people with no understanding of what is occurring. It is a state in which raw aggression and aggressive tendencies are ever-present. Thinking is distorted and action without thought predominates; in other words, action replaces thought (Klein, 1946).

In discussing the paranoid-schizoid position, Klein (1946) also described the infant's need to mentally erase aspects of the self that are threatening to his or her sense of security, aspects that are too much to bear. In the paranoid-schizoid position, anxiety is intense because the projector fears persecution for what he or she has expelled onto another.

When movement or growth occurs, however, when aggression and other unbearable feelings are modulated, modified, or made tolerable in some manner, the way of experiencing the self and others shifts. In this second state or way of relating to the world, the position Klein (1946) called the "depressive position" (not to be confused with clinical depression), feelings are "taken back" or reclaimed. They no longer have to be projected, but can be experienced as belonging to the self. Others are experienced as whole people, with various qualities and characteristics; some may be appreciated and some not, but good and bad qualities can coexist within the same person without one or more parts having to be eradicated or disavowed. In this position, opportunities for mourning, repair, and learning from past experience become possible. Thinking also emerges or is restored in this state. This process of change occurs in the context of a relational world wherein one's initial raw aggression is modified and made bearable with the help of another or others.

Although Klein's (1946) ideas were originally conceptualized as a way to describe how children develop intrapsychically, they were later woven into her understanding of adult patients. Today they are used as they were originally conceived, and have also been elaborated upon by various people to describe how groups of people interact (e.g. Bion, 1962). This includes infant and mother dyads, reigning rulers and their people, patient and therapist pairs, as well as couples and families. Other theorists, for example Donald Meltzer (1973) and C. Fred Alford (1989), have used these concepts to describe aspects of internal terror and social theory.

Since Kleinian concepts have evolved to include many situations and now have wide-ranging appeal in terms of describing the human condition, I believe their application should be considered when thinking about all interactions that are perceived as having gone awry, whether they be interpersonal exchanges, historical, recent political developments, or global issues of war. When communication between two people or among many breaks down, or has not occurred at all, varying degrees of difficulty ranging from simple misunderstanding to massive acts of terror can result as individuals or groups of people rid themselves of negative feelings. They then project these feelings onto others and proceed by navigating in the world as if the original feelings emanated from another or others in the first place. This in turn provides justification for the projector(s) to engage in violence against the perceived enemy or enemies, whether in thoughts, words, or deeds. Hence, while many factors are involved in conflict of any type, I believe the mechanism of projective identification is a major component of the process. When any type of revenge or crime or heinous act of terror against another is committed, either by one individual against another or by one group against another group, projection of some form of aggression that cannot be tolerated rears its ugly head.

To further elaborate on the aggression and aggressive tendencies inherent in all of us, it is worth considering certain aspects of Newton's Laws of Thermodynamics and Einstein's later interpretation of them. Extrapolating from and incorporating the essence of the idea that energy can neither be created nor destroyed, but only modified (Newton's First Law of Thermodynamics), one might reasonably postulate that the same theory applies to aggression. Whether we are born with it, as many theorists believe, or whether it emerges as part of normal development as we encounter inevitable frustrations and disappointments in life, aggression is part of the human condition. It is within each of us as long as we are alive and does not simply disappear; for like energy or, perhaps more aptly stated, as a *form* of energy, it cannot be destroyed, but only modulated or modified in some way. Assuming that raw aggression does exist within all of us, then it must be converted to a more palatable form to be experienced, contained, understood within, and then used productively. If this transformation does not happen, violence against the self or others can occur in a myriad of ways, including the infliction of pain and terror upon people since, as is the case with energy, aggression does not simply disappear.

Since Klein's time, further development of this psychoanalytic phenomenon has emerged, and it is through the lens of these advancements that I analyze what happened to the women, and groups of women, whose stories I tell. Violence was done to their emotions, their character, and their very psyches. Historically, this has been at the hands of men and groups of men, because men have been in positions of power for the most part. Why, in addition to the cultural prejudices I suggest, have men treated women with such aggression? What was it about their own experiences that has permitted men to act in the ways they have, and why have women accepted their behavior? And what hope exists for remedying the damage that has been done? I provide explanations of the processes involved in projective identification as well as illustrations, usually from my private practice, of these concepts as they emerge in everyday life. I also discuss how projections can be taken back and the benefits that can ensue from this action.

Expansion of the concept; others add to the definition

From another, similar perspective, Otto Kernberg contrasted projection with projective identification: "Projective identification is seen as an early or primitive defense operation, [while] projection [is] later or more advanced and derivative in nature." Nevertheless, "the operation of [projective identification has] ... cognitive preconditions" (1987, p. 795). In projective identification, the projector believes that the object or recipient is transformed, or at least altered by—"identified" with—the negative fantasy he or she has projected. He then behaves toward the recipient as if his projected, despised self has been internalized by its object and is "true" (Kernberg, 1987).

In this classical view, the object (or victim) of projection is not considered separately; in practice, moreover, the object is almost always the analyst. Early writers sometimes used the term "introjection" to characterize the effect on the object. Others noted the connection of projective identification to psychoanalytic "splitting" (Grotstein, 1981).

A more recent distinction deserves mention, since it is based on an ambiguity within the original theory of projective identification: Does the object of the projection "receive" it or even know about it (a "two-body" situation), or can she or he be unaware of the unconscious fantasy (a "one-body" situation), as Klein (1946) believed? This issue is well delineated by John Zinner (2001), who turns to Kernberg (1987) to define the "two-body" process: The patient projects the intolerable onto an object and maintains a connection to what has been projected, thereafter "attempting to control the object as a continuation of the defensive efforts against the intolerable intrapsychic experience, and ... unconsciously inducing in the object what is projected in the actual interactions with the object" (Zinner, 2001, pp. 7–8). "Projective identification does not exist where there is no interaction between projector and recipient" (Ogden, 1982, p. 14). The distinction may turn on the question of who is "identifying" with the ugly fantasy-person: the projector (one-body) or the recipient (two-body), subject or object.

Zinner (2001), as a practicing psychiatrist, argues for the one-body view in which the patient both projects his hostile fantasy and identifies with it as part of his image of the recipient. The latter does not perceive some mysterious Doppelgänger within herself, but recognizes the situation only by the behavior of the projector. Following Kernberg's (1987) proposal, Zinner (2001) suggests a set of developmental stages in the functioning of projective identification, no longer limited to the hallucinations and delusions of psychotic or borderline personalities, or even to the analytic situation. "It seems to me common sense that projective identification must be a ubiquitous phenomenon which is not limited to the psychoses and severe character disorders" (p. 15), but is utilized as a defense in neurosis, in transference, and in normal emotional conflicts. Some of this latter activity, Zinner concedes, could be called simple "projection." The projector with these less-severe problems can usually be helped to clarify the self-other boundary, to acknowledge and reinternalize the projection, and to modify the distortion and regain a realistic image of the recipient. My own practice encourages me to concur.

But Zinner (2001) wishes to extend the definition of projective identification still further, into a conscious mental activity in which defensive needs to externalize no longer significantly influence the construction of the object image. The subject is, in a probing fashion, temporarily loosening the self-object boundary in an effort to find a resonance in his own experience with what his senses are telling him about the external object.

When following Zinner's (2001) thinking as stated above, the projector is merely trying to understand another person, to "approximate the actuality of the other" (p. 18). Thus, according to Zinner, one form of projective identification is empathy—the capacity to put oneself in another's shoes. It describes a process of the conscious mind. From this perspective we create our own versions of people based on who we are, who they are, and what we make of who they are at any given moment in time, a useful concept and one that differs from the defensive use of projective identification.

It is clear that various definitions of this concept can help us better understand the ways in which people interact, keep others at an arm's length, unconsciously damage the other, or simply communicate.

Working with a powerful unconscious force: illustrations of despair and the emergence of hope

In my work I primarily use the concept of projective identification as a way of understanding and explaining how the suffering patient experiences these "transfers of feelings" from others as they receive powerful and unwanted states of mind defensively inflicted upon them by another. The possibility of the projected-upon person identifying with the projection is one outcome that can emerge from the process, making this a two-body phenomenon. In my view, based on clinical experience, the projector is likely to retain some of the expelled fantasy in his or her own sense of self, but not to genuinely identify with it until he or she has worked through conflicts that emerge in relation to psychic pain.

Although Klein (1946) eventually wove her theory into her understanding of adult patients, her ideas were originally conceptualized as a way to describe how children develop intrapsychically. From this perspective, all babies are born in the paranoid-schizoid position. Although they can begin to move toward the depressive position when they realize they are separate beings, there is always a movement back to the original position at times of vulnerability.

Think, for example, of a two-year-old child I once saw with her family and who was bitten by a younger sibling in my office during their session. A natural response for the bitten child, who did not understand that sometimes babies bite to ease the pain of teething, was to get angry. Perhaps the toddler was already holding unbearable feelings of jealousy and rage after the birth of her sibling. Lacking an explanation for his aggressive action, her only recourse seemed to be to damage the baby, kicking, screaming at, or hitting the new arrival who had injured her. Meanwhile, the teething baby initially did not know he was hurting his sibling, and now was hurt himself and did not seem to understand why.

Until the mother consoled and explained, the two-year-old was filled with anger that couldn't be understood or tolerated. She would run and sit on her mother's lap, proclaiming, "The baby bit me, but I didn't do anything." At this point in her young life, she thought the new baby was bad and should be punished. But mother, who was most often focusing on what was going on in the room, would say, "Annie, you are the big sister; go help your brother, he's just a baby." The young child could not process what I imagined she felt: unconscious fear of abandonment and loss of love from her mother. She appeared to be emotionally devastated.

If this scene were repeated many times without a caregiver speaking with either child, tension would likely escalate, with both children building up resentment and anger. If these feelings were never dealt with, various negative results could follow, from the emergence of physical fighting to the development of sadomasochistic tendencies—with neither child ever grasping the underpinnings of their hostility toward the other. Even such small infractions, when they are not mediated by a caregiver, are likely to cause negative feelings, possibly for a lifetime. When a subsequent negative event occurs, one or both siblings could blame the other by denying responsibility, always claiming the other is at fault.

But if the mother or caregiver had the sensitivity to accept and contain each child's sense of anger and hostility while holding onto these emotions and benevolently transforming them to calmness by her soothing manner, the world could be a safe place again. The baby could sense his mother's understanding and thereafter his feelings of confidence and safety could be rebuilt. His temporary projection could be on the wane; he might well be able to move forward. The toddler could gradually learn to describe her feelings to her mother, who could help her process them. Obviously, this view of projective identification and its consequences goes far beyond the closed analytic situation into the world of experience: the daily life of everyday families. Some naturally know how to cope with these encounters and some do not, which can set the stage for hostile and aggressive feelings among family members.

Another example of projection identification can be seen in a patient whom I shall call John. A number of years ago, John had a brief affair with the woman of his dreams, whom I shall refer to as Alison, a woman with whom he had had a long-standing friendship. In therapy John claimed to desperately want and need a "perfect" person like Alison, stating that his wife was an aggressive woman who only cared about her work. After a year-long email and phone relationship with this "ideal" woman who had been very flirtatious, provocative, and seductive, often stating that she longed to leave her husband for him, they met and shared one romantic evening culminating in "the most tender, best sexual experience either had ever had" (in John's description). After that evening, they vowed to find a way to be together.

Shortly thereafter, however, Alison wrote one short email saying that John had misunderstood her, and that she did not wish to be in contact with him ever again. My patient was devastated, briefly blamed himself, and initially stated that the entire incident had been his fault from the beginning. Alison, on the other hand, he exonerated from any culpability. John steadfastly maintained her innocence, claiming that she personified goodness and "the saintliness of an angel."

As this perplexing picture continued to unfold, the focus of John's feelings about his participation in the events leading up to the affair began to shift as I became, in his eyes, inept, not helpful, and generally of little use to him, i.e. I became the "bad" one. He said I was disingenuous and was only interested in payment of my fees. Despite my many attempts to interpret and help him understand what had occurred with Alison and what was happening between us, one month of subtle dissatisfaction with me turned into many months of more blatant denigration of my thoughts and ideas.

At that point, John started to talk about looking for another type of therapy. He said he needed something more "proactive," continuing to maintain Alison's goodness while highlighting my lack of understanding and uselessness. In this case, this patient could not deal with the aggression he felt toward Alison, projected it onto me, and planned to exit so he would not have to deal with the unbearable anger and hatred he felt toward her, on top of the emotional pain he initially experienced from her rejection. This is an effective example of the paranoid-schizoid position, wherein Alison could not be understood as a whole person, but rather was idealized and protected from my patient's disappointment, sadness, and wrath.

It is also an example of distorted thinking wherein (without fully understanding what had occurred) John wanted to take action by finding another therapist who would not remind him of his wretched feelings. Unconsciously, I believe he also wanted me to feel what it was like to be abandoned, hence his wish to leave an analysis that had previously been important to him. And so he projected Alison's betrayal (and his denial of it) onto me. Thanks to my training and long clinical practice with such patients, I was able to ward off identification with his negative opinion of my treatment. This experience helped me understand that protective identification is a primitive protection, a shield for warding off an intolerable feeling, such as rejection by the beloved, by pushing it away.

Another example of projective identification

Moving to the current landscape of our political world and the 2016 presidential election campaign, we can see a very public exhibition of projective identification in action. Now, in an attempt to better demonstrate how hostile actions from bullying to terrorism come to occur, it is useful to consider the candidates and the surly and aggressive behavior we saw from them up to election day. These candidates could have successfully negotiated their differences in a world where thinking prevailed, but they failed to do so because unconscious forces were at play. They attributed to others what they could not tolerate within, thus wreaking havoc on those onto whom the aggression was directed. If the recipients of such "balls of badness" had been able to make a secure connection with their opponents, perhaps the debates would not have been so acrimonious. The candidates might have been able to recover from the pain that projections caused. With effective communication, respect, and understanding the other's right to dissent, even the aggressors may have been able to maintain a sense of dignity. The concept of "one-body" projective identification is also highly useful, particularly in the context of the stories of women I've described. I do not limit the function of projection to the two-person description.

The dreadful situations I describe do not require that the object(s) or recipient(s) of anger, hostility, or humiliation absorb into their own psyche the negative emotions, conscious or unconscious, that are projected their way. These unfortunate women might not even recognize what is happening. Sometimes it is not clear, without specific information, whether projective identification is of a one-body or two-body type, since it is necessary to know how the projector experienced the projection before determining the category of this mechanism. An example of projective identification recently appeared in *The Times* through an interview with a renowned psychiatrist, John Zinner, warning that we all are facing an existential crisis due to Trump's self-appointed right to launch a nuclear weapon anytime for any reason he deems appropriate (May 20, 2017). Zinner, a psychiatrist and clinical professor at George Washington University, argues that the rule against speaking publicly about the psyches of public figures is superseded by a broader duty to society.

In the article, Trump is described as having a type of character consisting of a fundamental self-esteem issue coupled with grandiosity. One aspect of this character is expressed in his tendency to call people names. After dismissing James Comey, Trump referred to him as a "grandstander" and a "showboat." Other names he has lobbed at those who've fallen out of favor with him are "weak," "failure," "liar," and "loser." But these names are nothing other than projected images of traits he is unable to tolerate within himself; what we see at work here is projective identification.

This article highlights the mechanism that is so pervasively present in the destruction of the other, whether it be a person, people in a group, or countries. Nevertheless, in this situation we do not know how it affected Comey personally, so we cannot say it was a one-body or two-body phenomenon. On the one hand, it might have been devastating to him and he might have believed that there was something to the negative things Trump said, making it a two-body process. On the other hand, he might have "considered the source" while thinking the President was just doing what he frequently does when he is angry: He says whatever comes to him without filtering his thoughts. He could, after all, have waited to talk with his attorney to determine whether or not his ideas or notions could be appropriately disclosed to reporters on television. He could have kept them to himself until he figured out how to handle this situation in an appropriate manner.

Projective identification can affect groups of people as well as individuals. In fact, with groups, the possibility of "identification" with the projection may make their punishing activities more vicious, because their colleagues are watching.

As pessimistic as this scenario might seem, Melanie Klein (1946) does not doom people—projectors or anyone else—to live forever in the despair of the paranoid-schizoid position. Some, projectors as well as recipients, do emerge, as the examples of the teething baby and John demonstrate. She posits a second position: the depressive position. When aggression and other unbearable feelings can be modulated, modified, or made tolerable in some manner, the way of experiencing the self and others can shift. Movement or growth can occur. This second way of relating to the world permits intensely hostile feelings to be understood, reclaimed or "taken back." They no longer have to be projected, but can be experienced as belonging to the self and are subdued. Others are now experienced as whole people, with various qualities and characteristics. Some of the qualities of these others may be appreciated and some not, but the person in the depressed position realizes that good and bad characteristics may coexist in the same person without one part having to be eradicated or disavowed. In this position, opportunities for mourning, repair, and learning from past experience become possible. Rational thinking is also restored.

With the help of another or others, the process of change occurs in the context of a relational world wherein one's initial raw aggression is modified and made bearable. Different terms have been used by Klein (1946) and her followers to describe this process, most notably by Wilfred Bion (1962), who called it "containment" and the "alpha process." If it is successful, aggression in any of its forms is transformed so that it becomes a new aspect of the self.

References

Alford, C. F. (1989). *Melanie Klein and critical social theory: An account of politics, art, and reason based on her psychoanalytic theory*. Chelsea: Bookcrafters, Inc.

Bion, W. R. (1962). *Learning from experience*. London: Heinemann. Reprinted in paper by Maresfield Reprints. London: Karnac Books.

Grotstein, J. (1981). *Splitting and projective identification*. Northvale, NJ: Jason Aronson.

Kernberg, O. (1987). Projection and projective identification: Developmental and clinical aspects. *Journal of the American Psychanalytic Association, 35*, 795–819.

Klein, M. (1946). Notes on some schizoid mechanisms. *International Journal of Psychoanalysis, 27*, 99–110.

Meltzer, D. (1973). *Sexual states of mind*. London: Karnac Books Ltd.

Messina, K. (2009). Taking back projections: The despair and hope in projective identification. Paper presented at 2nd Annual International Conference on the Human Condition, Barrie, Ontario, May 2008. Published in *Engaging terror: A critical and interdisciplinary approach*, ed. Marianne Vardalos. Boca Raton, FL: Universal Publishers, Inc./BrownWalker Press.

Ogden, T. H. (1982). *Projective identification and therapeutic technique*. New York: Jason Aronson.

Pavia, W. (2017). The psychiatrists' verdict: Donald Trump is a man incapable of guilt, with inner rage. *The Times*, May 20, n.p.

Spillius, E. (2007). *Encounters with Melanie Klein*. London and New York: Routledge.

Zinner, J. (2001). A developmental spectrum of projective identification, pp. 28–34. In Proceedings of the International Conference of the Society of Psychoanalytical Marital Psychotherapists. Oxford, UK, Society of Psychoanalytical Marital Psychotherapists.

2

CLARA THOMPSON'S DISAPPEARANCE

How projective identification contributed to the near-extinction of a star

The story begins

Among the many historical paradigm shifts that have occurred in Washington, DC, the advancement of psychoanalysis was no exception. In the first half of the 20th century, psychiatrists and psychologists as well as people from other disciplines and various cultural backgrounds came together to develop what would eventually become a two-person psychology. This development was different from Freud's one-person psychology, which gave power to the all-knowing analyst of intrapsychic processes, who focused primarily on interpreting conflict.

Much thinking about this new way of treating patients, i.e., through the curative effect of "the relationship," occurred at Chestnut Lodge in Bethesda, MD, and at St. Elizabeth Hospital in Washington, DC, as well as at Sheppard and Enoch Pratt Hospital near Baltimore, where Harry Stack Sullivan worked with psychotic patients in new ways. Many more innovative ideas emerged at the Washington School of Psychiatry (WSP). Widely respected as an interdisciplinary training facility for a variety of specialties, it was officially founded in 1936 (Taylor, 2009).

The new group of innovative thinkers and practitioners at these locations became known as "the interpersonalists." Their combined knowledge was the bedrock on which relational theories were built, theories that play a major role in current psychoanalytic and psychodynamic schools of thought. As important as this work was to the field, key members of the group, composed of Sullivan, Clara Thompson, Erich Fromm, and Frieda Fromm-Reichmann, have received little credit in the annals of history.

Clara Thompson in particular has gone largely unnoticed, or at least has been pushed to the margins. While she was a classically trained psychoanalyst, she was also able to look at most theoretical writing in a balanced way. She used what she thought was still viable in older contributions while working toward integrating newer ideas. Being true to her own thoughts, she wrote variations of or added to some of Freud's ideas. This was not easy because of the criticism she got from some of the European-trained Freudians who came to America to escape World War II, and who thought of themselves as the only true psychoanalysts. Yet Thompson soldiered on, writing 57 publications in her lifetime. To a few current theorists she was very important. According to Mitchell and Black (1995), Clara Thompson was the person most responsible for shaping interpersonal psychoanalysis in its contemporary form. Yet her legacy is all but extinct. In this book I ask, and hope to answer, how and why this erasure happened.

Who was Clara Thompson?

Said to be a spunky woman who stood up for what she believed in, for herself, her colleagues, and friends, Clara Thompson blazed a rocky trail during tough times to make it easier for all of us. However, for the most part, very few people have heard of her. She was not only a true pioneer but also a wavemaker who set the stage for women of future generations by standing up for her beliefs. According to Erich Fromm, who knew her very well, Clara Thompson could not be intimidated. He also indicated that she was trustworthy, had integrity, and was reliable. Her loyalty to friends was also said to be one of her outstanding traits (Green, 1964).

Ferenczi and Budapest

By the 1920s, Clara Thompson was already a well-trained psychiatrist and psychoanalyst who was thoroughly familiar with the teachings of Freud. She also knew Harry Stack Sullivan. However, she did not know much about Sándor Ferenczi, a Hungarian psychoanalyst. One day while meeting with Sullivan in Washington, she mentioned that she was looking for a new psychoanalyst and asked Sullivan for a recommendation. He suggested Ferenczi and encouraged her to go to Budapest to be analyzed by him (Taylor, 2009).

After a brief meeting with Ferenczi at a conference in New York and based on her initial impression of him as well as her wish to be in treatment with a forward-thinking analyst, Thompson spent two summers in Budapest as Ferenczi's student, beginning in 1928. She then moved there and became his analysand until his unexpected death in 1933 (in Budapest in 1928, analytic candidates were students of their analyst before becoming patients). Prior to making the transition from the Baltimore-Washington area to Budapest, Thompson made an agreement with Sullivan: Once she returned from Budapest, she would share with him what she had learned from Ferenczi (Taylor, 2009).

Ultimately, Clara Thompson's work with Ferenczi changed the course of history. What she shared about her experiences had a major impact on Sullivan. In fact, according to Taylor (2009), Sullivan counted what he learned from Clara Thompson's work with Ferenczi as one of the major influences in his life. What Thompson herself learned was particularly important at that point in history because she was able to talk and write about Ferenczi's ideas and practices, whereas Ferenczi himself had to keep most of his theories and techniques to himself in order to stay in Freud's good graces. The price he paid was that his work remained obscure for some time. Up until 1988, when his diaries were published, he was not a household name, primarily because he deviated from Freud so much (Taylor, 2009).

We now know there was an undeniable link between what was developing in Central Europe in the burgeoning field of psychoanalytic thinking and what was occurring in Washington in the late '20s, although much of the latter activity was not widely known or acknowledged at the time (Taylor, 2009). Yet many of Sullivan's most prominent theories emerged from Clara Thompson's analysis with Sándor Ferenczi. Her experience, much of which she shared with Sullivan, added to his concept of the shifting role of the therapist in the participant-observer relationship. Hence, Thompson's generous sharing of ideas and willingness to talk about much of her experience with Ferenczi, as well as her part in preserving much of his work, speaks for itself (Messina, 2014). However, there are naysayers who dismiss her contributions, a phenomenon that will be explored in this book.

Clara Thompson's contributions, leadership, and her critics

Lewis Aron (2001), a well-respected relational psychoanalyst, has credited Thompson with being the driving force behind the contemporary interpersonal school of thought. In an earlier work of mine I drew a similar conclusion. Clara Thompson kept Ferenczi's work relevant by sharing what she learned from him with her colleagues when she returned to America after his death in 1933 (Messina, 2014).

Clara Thompson's contributions helped make today's psychoanalytic questions answerable. The popular relational school of the 1990s mentioned previously exists because Thompson brought Ferenczi's work to America. She dedicated much of her life to furthering the understanding of this new breed of psychoanalysis wherein the relationship is the curative factor.

Unfortunately, while the early relationalists drew upon Ferenczi's wisdom, they seem to have forgotten their "mother" and skilled communicator who kept Ferenczi's thinking alive. While they quote and adulate Ferenczi frequently, Thompson is almost never cited in their writing—even their historical writing. Why has Thompson been excluded from an important place on the relationalists' ancestral family tree?

Another contribution that Thompson made was her effort to promote the psychological differences between women and men. Ruth Moulton (1986) has said that Thompson was the first American woman who wrote about the psychology of women in six articles and a book in the 1940s and early '50s, a period when even raising the question of the individuality of women was to risk criticism and censure.

According to Moulton (1986), Clara Thompson spoke clearly in her own voice; she was not simply an interpreter of others. Her observations were lucid and pragmatic. In "Penis Envy in Woman" Thompson (Green, 1964) was referring to a type of envy in a symbolic way. She was not talking about envy of male anatomy but rather was referring to the advantages men had (and still have) in our society. She also talked about female sexuality in its own right, not in terms of wishing for a penis but instead referring to inhibitions caused by cultural restrictions. While these ideas are commonplace today, according to Moulton (1986) in the 1940s and '50s they were new ideas that raised cultural issues facing women during that period in history.

In the 1950s Clara Thompson also taught these new ideas about women in Western culture, with great success, to students at the Washington School of Psychiatry and the William Alanson White Institute. On April 21, 1952, while executive director of the William Alanson White Institute in New York City, Thompson wrote a letter to "Duke" (Captain Theodore) Dukeshire of the Washington School of Psychiatry agreeing to give a seminar on the psychology of women. She recommended that participants be limited to psychologists, psychiatrists, and social workers, with no more than 20 students in the class. Thompson included a course description in which she proposed to "evaluate the psychoanalytic concepts of the psychology of women." She further proposed to discuss how a woman's psychology is affected by physiological and biological factors and how her development is shaped by cultural attitudes.

On December 8, 1952, Dukeshire wrote a letter to Thompson soliciting her insights about "the school" and its future, suggesting that they discuss the matter over lunch on December 13. In the letter he said, "Thank you for arranging to have the contributions to be sent down" and predicted that at three dollars apiece it would have many eager takers. Dukeshire additionally told Thompson that he had "heard many fine comments" from students in regard to her course, The Psychology of Women.

While Karen Horney, Helene Deutsch, and others are widely recognized by contemporary feminist psychologists and psychoanalysts, the name Clara Thompson is rarely mentioned, even though she wrote about women's issues and taught courses that were well received. Her ideas about the differences between men and women have mostly been superseded by feminist theory and psychological research of the 1970s and beyond, but in most disciplines, feminists honor their foremothers. In Clara Thompson's case, that didn't really happen.

Major obstacles that led to her veil of invisibility

One question seems obvious: If her work was so transformative, at least on paper and probably in practice, why has Clara Thompson been largely forgotten?

A half-century after her major contributions were published, much of the work of Clara Thompson was attacked by two analysts who never knew her, attacks that I believe contributed to her erasure.

Susan Shapiro (1993) and B. William Brennan (2015) resurrected stories about Thompson's experiences with Ferenczi that ridiculed her based on tenaciously held ideas that seem to me to lack clear evidence. And their tone is unnecessary, as rancor of any degree is uncalled for based on the nature of the criticism. Of course, there are always skeptics who dissect the creations of others rather than building on structures of their own to add to a community of ideas; however, the specific focus and virulence with which these two write strikes me as a bit odd given all that is possible to select from in our field today concerning Clara Thompson.

They both appeared to place a great deal of emphasis on Ferenczi's personal notes that he never intended to make public. One of their major hypotheses is based on an entry in Ferenczi's diary (Dupont, 1988), which references the case of his patient "Dm.," a lady who, "complying with my passivity, had allowed herself to take more and more liberties, and occasionally even kissed me" (Dupont, 1988, p. 2). Ferenczi went on to say that this behavior met with no resistance (on his part): "I first reacted to the unpleasantness that ensued with the complete impassivity with which I was conducting this analysis" (p. 2). Based on this self-report, one wonders why Thompson was so harshly criticized for telling a fellow student about her analysis with Ferenczi (Brennan, 2015).

With regard to Sue Shapiro, a powerful example of a destructive critique can be found in her article "Ferenczi's Messenger with Half a Message" (Shapiro, 1993). Essentially, Shapiro claims that Clara Thompson was sexually abused as a child by her father, that she undoubtedly discussed the abuse with Ferenczi in her analysis and that, when she presented his work to her American colleagues after she left Budapest in 1933, she neglected to mention what Shapiro claims was Ferenczi's great interest in child sexual abuse. Thus, according to Shapiro, Thompson greatly harmed the development of psychoanalytic theory by misrepresenting or neglecting to focus on Ferenczi's theory of childhood sexual abuse in her communications with the American psychoanalytic community.

Shapiro's (Shapiro, 1993) annoyance with Thompson appears to have called into question her veracity as a writer. By admonishing Thompson for not lecturing about Ferenczi's ideas of sexual abuse once she had returned to the United States, she has failed to mentalize in two ways: First, she cannot have known what was on Clara Thompson's mind in 1933. Second, saying what Thompson "should" have done more than a half-century earlier when the tenor of the culture was very different is altogether unfair. Why did Shapiro not allow Thompson to have her own experience? Why would Thompson have had the same thoughts as Shapiro when people were not openly talking about child abuse almost 80 years ago? Shapiro is talking about *her* interest in sexual abuse, not Clara Thompson's interest. Moreover, why did Thompson have a specific charge to disseminate Ferenczi's thinking about children?

In addition to initially accusing Thompson of causing damage to the field of psychoanalysis by failing to discuss Ferenczi's ideas about childhood sexual abuse, Shapiro changed her argument, later implying that Thompson *might not* have been abused after all, saying that even if she weren't abused, she should have "spread the word when she returned to America about the reality of abuse and its impact on children's lives" (Shapiro, 1993, p. 162). When you strongly support one side of an argument, even though you have no direct knowledge of anything associated with it, perhaps it is best to stay with that side of the discussion in order to mitigate confusion.

All things considered, assuming someone *should have* said something a half-century earlier is not logical. To reiterate, people were not talking freely about sexual abuse in 1933. As one gleans from Gelles (1993), one of the first times child abuse was acknowledged in print in this country was in 1962. That was more than 30 years after Thompson returned from Budapest. Even if the story were true, perhaps Thompson repressed the memory or maybe she was still experiencing the effects of trauma. If it were not true, and Eugene Taylor (2009), a well-respected scholar and expert in the history of psychoanalysis, was correct, it is gossip, hearsay, and the spreading of false information (more about Taylor's scholarly review of Thompson's life to follow). At any rate, it is not good scholarship to attempt to turn hypotheses into facts without evidence. Perhaps the words of Charles Dickens (1861) accurately depict a good rule for writers of historic figures. "Take nothing on its looks; take everything on evidence. There's no better rule" (*Great Expectations*, p. 40.19).

Some Ferenczi enthusiasts today essentially claim he was caught up in an enactment with Thompson but once he realized it, he apologized. Thereafter they indicate that Thompson was able to experience her mentor as someone different from her father, which allowed her to forgive him. While this interpretation sounds reasonable if one were sitting with a patient in 2018 or 2019, one must remember that Ferenczi was looking through a different lens in the '20s and '30s; "enactment" wasn't even a term that was used. "The term 'enactment' has only recently emerged as a technical one in psychoanalysis" (Aron & Harris, 2010, p. 18).

Unfortunately, Ferenczi's remarks about this segment of the analysis have been memorialized by some but seem inconclusive at best. By today's standards one might say Ferenczi's conclusion was a bit of a leap, as was his statement about Thompson's behavior at a social event.

> But then the patient began to make herself ridiculous, ostentatiously as it were, in her sexual conduct (for example at social gatherings, while dancing). It was only through the insight and admission that my passivity had been unnatural that she was brought back to real life, so to speak, as insight does have to reckon with social opposition. Simultaneously, it became evident that here again was a case of repression of the father-child situation. As a child, Dm. had been grossly abused sexually by her father,

who was out of control; later, obviously because of the father's bad conscience and social anxiety, he reviled her, so to speak. The daughter had to take revenge on her father indirectly, by failing in her own life.
(Dupont, 1988, p. 2)

With regard to this quote by Ferenczi reported by Dupont (1988), I wonder how "she [referring to Thompson] began to make herself 'ridiculous'" (p. 2)? This statement would need to be described before it could be seriously considered. Also, would this have been said of a male patient? I doubt it. Furthermore, what Ferenczi claimed was "obvious" was not. While it may have been somewhat clear to him, it is not to the reader—although one cannot blame Ferenczi for that, since it was not his intention to expose his private notes. Perhaps those who chose to publish this material might have considered more thoroughly the impact of their zeal to bring it into the public eye. Ferenczi's notes were never intended to be shared with millions of people. It's a wonder people today aren't nervous about this type of thing happening again. I find myself wondering if Balint, who intended to publish the private notes of patients for years, or Dupont, who did publish them, would have agreed to have their own analyses published after their deaths. I also wonder if Shapiro and Brennan would agree to have their analyses scrutinized by psychoanalysts.

While Sándor Ferenczi had theoretical ideas and ways of working that changed the whole course of psychoanalytic thinking, regrettably these major contributions may not be found in his diary (Dupont, 1988). Yet many of his notions in the above paragraphs seem to have been "cast in stone" and believed by at least some of his admirers as if they are irrefutable truths. This is in spite of the fact that speculating and making interpretations based on what one gleans from Ferenczi's diary (Dupont, 1988), which was never meant to be a comprehensive summation of his thinking, is not the best way to thoroughly understand what Ferenczi had to offer. Fragments of sentences and personal information about patients that was not written for publication (people were sometimes referred to in the feminine form and sometimes in the masculine form, with different initials used in various places) is not evidence of anything. Nor is it an example of scholarly research.

In addition, Ferenczi's definition of the sexual abuse, which may be known to only a few who have access to the unpublished papers of Clara Thompson, is complicated since Ferenczi had more than one definition of childhood trauma as it relates to sexuality: One type of abuse was physically perpetrated by the parent *upon* the child, and another was subtler and did not involve physicality but related to a fantasy.

> In the unpublished section of *Thompson's Evaluation of Ferenczi's Relaxation Therapy*, which was written in 1933, Thompson gives a much closer account of Ferenczi's ideas: "It is possible that the trauma is not necessarily of a gross sexual nature, but on the more subtle nature of the reaction of

the child to parental erotic tensions and guilt ... the child does not suffer from their own Oedipal complex but from that of the parents" (*Thompson Papers*, 1933, pp. 17–18)

(Brennan, 2015, p. 93)

This leads one to wonder what type of abuse Ferenczi was referring to when speaking of Clara Thompson. It is also curious that something so seemingly important was omitted from Thompson's published work. To cast further doubt on the diary (Dupont, 1988), it is important to consider that, while some people loved Clara Thompson, others were ambivalent and still others may have disliked her. In any event, I haven't ever read anywhere that she "failed in life." When Ferenczi wrote, "The daughter had to take revenge on her father indirectly, by failing in her own life," (p. 3) was he referring to Clara Thompson? Or, was this an example of his use of a coding system wherein he tried to elaborate on and study his patient's character traits (he talked about several patients in the same paragraph, which sometimes made it hard to know to whom he was referring)? Furthermore, since Ferenczi went to so much trouble to disguise the patients in his diary and presumably wrote notes for his own personal information, perhaps his way of recording and analyzing information about his patients was more complex than anyone knew. He also, as mentioned above, would sometimes refer to the same patient using a masculine pronoun and a feminine one interchangeably, and would write about a single patient using inconsistent initials (Dupont, 1988). Why would he do that? Certainly there was a method to his system, but only he knew its logic. One example of many arbitrary changes is described on page 37 (Dupont, 1988). "The patient in the passage, R.N. is a woman. In the diary Ferenczi sometimes uses masculine pronouns to refer to her; for the sake of clarity we have changed these to the feminine gender." Why would anyone do this? Ferenczi had a conscious or unconscious reason for describing patients the way he did. Why not wonder about this phenomenon, a much more psychoanalytic way of processing information, rather than simply changing words?

The fact that the patients in the diary were identified in the first place raises questions. Why was this done by his students and admirers after Ferenczi went to so much trouble to disguise his patients? As noted by Shapiro (1993, p. 162), perhaps the patients were identified in retaliation because Thompson told one of Freud's analysands that Ferenczi allowed her to kiss him.

It is also possible, as various people who knew him have indicated, that Ferenczi was impaired when he wrote close to the time of his death in 1933, by "mental deterioration" as Jones suggested (Dupont, 1988, p. xix). With regard to possible impairment, Dupont's book (1988) brought to light another question about Ferenczi's state of mind. According to Dupont (1988), Ferenczi's wife said he sometimes read the newspaper upside-down, a curious habit for someone whom Dupont claims was of sound mind. Dupont also said, "In the entry on July 15 he says he is schizophrenic, delusional, paranoid, emotionally vacant, managing to function only by overcompensating for all he lacks" (Dupont, 1988, p. xxiv). Given this self-assessment of his state of mind, which indicated he was having trouble with thinking clearly, it is interesting to note that Dupont seemed to disregard this information. Dupont was only eight years old at the time of Ferenczi's death and could not have known about his state of mind, yet she suggested he was thinking clearly in spite of the fact that he said something to the contrary. "In any case ... this caricature, accounts for a great ability to achieve distance from himself and with remarkable lucidity, rather than mental disintegration, as Jones wanted to believe and to make others believe" (p. xxiv). Hence, Dupont's endorsement of Ferenczi's writing style proves nothing. Based on today's standards, it is not good form to analyze someone's state of mind without having actually known and worked with that person.

Another thing worth considering is Ferenczi's earlier way of navigating in the world that troubled Freud (Dupont, 1988). When being admonished by Freud in the famous December 13 letter for his "Kissing Technique," Freud inserted a reproach to Ferenczi for his pre-analytic tendency for sexual play with patients,

> according to my recollection a tendency to sex play with patients was not completely alien to you in pre-analytic times, so that new technique could be linked to an old error. That is why I spoke in my last letter of a new puberty.
>
> *(Dupont, 1988, pp. 3–4)*

Hence it is no surprise that some of these "patient's issues" were related to Ferenczi's psychology. Although he had engaged in inappropriate sexual behavior with patients previously, only Freud seemed to be concerned. Dupont, Shapiro, Balint, and Brennan did not seem bothered by it, if silence on the matter of sexual indiscretion suggests lack of concern for such behavior.

As it turns out, there are additional questions about the translation of the diary. Dupont (1988), who was Balint's niece, knew about some of the idiosyncratic codes Ferenczi employed, but was satisfied with the translation, whereas Balint (Dupont, 1988), who did the translating, was not so convinced that everything was an accurate representation of Ferenczi's ideas. Although Balint held on to the diaries for more than 40 years and may have done a fine job preserving this work, who is to say that he knew all aspects of Ferenczi's coding system, which seems idiosyncratic to say the least? For the reason mentioned above, I believe there are still questions about the accuracy of everything stated about Ferenczi's patients in the diary.

Another problem arises because of Balint's decision to take out paragraphs that were damaging for men while apparently feeling free to put in everything and anything negative about a woman. Case in point: Balint (cited in Dupont, 1988) took out paragraphs written by Ferenczi that might have been offensive about Freud (p. viii), but left in things about "Dm." (Clara Thompson) that made her look sexually provocative, unstable, and even unclean. That was apparently okay in Balint's book: It's acceptable to disparage our founding mother, but we must protect our revered founding fathers. Why, one might wonder? Why is it OK to disparage women while protecting men?

Returning to Shapiro (1993), as mystifying as her need to denounce Thompson is in the first place, it is equally perplexing to read the way in which she seems to defend her in the last paragraph of her paper.

> And, like many great women of her generation—Margaret Mead, Georgia O'Keeffe, Eleanor Roosevelt—Thompson kept her insecurities, longing, and need for comfort from other women closeted as well while working for a day when that would be unnecessary.
>
> *(Shapiro, 1993, p. 171)*

Of course, women in the 1920s and early '30s were not talking openly about their sexual abuse, that's not what people did more than 90 years ago. Why would Shapiro have had that expectation? Maybe it is her way of apologizing to Thompson, but it seems disingenuous. It seems more likely to me that Sue Shapiro is still angry with Clara Thompson for failing to fill the role of the analytic grandmother she had been seeking. That may explain why Shapiro continues to write about Thompson, as recently, in fact, as 2017.[1] It feels almost as though she has to work something out and writing is helping her to do so. That Clara Thompson was a real woman with strengths and weaknesses does not seem to temper Shapiro's harsh judgment. Yet how can one go back in time and presume to know why anyone did anything, much less with such certainty? How is it possible to understand someone else's experience or judge him or her based on today's standards, particularly when the source of information is so questionable? I think Adam Phillip made a good point in this regard when he suggested that no one knows with certainty what really happened in any situation, not even the actual participants. There can only be readings and accounts of events, not known truths (Brennan, 2015).

With regard to the reporting of sexual offenses, I find it particularly outrageous that Shapiro found fault with Thompson for not wanting to report abuse that she heard from a patient in the 1950s when various male analysts blatantly had sex with patients and got away with it (Gabbard & Lester, 1994). Dr. G, for example, had sex with six women. Although he initially denied it, eventually he admitted it was true but refused to say he had done anything wrong and instead claimed it had helped the women. Instead of being expelled from his psychoanalytic institute, a supervisor rescued him. Unfortunately, men have gotten away with egregious acts against women then and they still do today. Fortunately, women have begun to fight back, and hopefully aren't blaming each other as Shapiro blamed Thompson (Shapiro, 1993). I wonder if she would have said a similar thing about a male therapist in the '50s. We won't know, but I suspect she wouldn't have done so, especially since it does not appear that she has to date. In my opinion, Sue Shapiro owes Clara Thompson an apology for being so insensitive by coming to the rescue of Ferenczi, who with his legion of fans hardly needs her support.

The fact that Shapiro (1993) has continued to question Clara Thompson's character is particularly distressing since she herself has admitted that one can't really say with certainty whether or not "Dm." was Clara Thompson (Shapiro, 1993). Additionally, it is most distressing that Shapiro casts aspersions on Thompson for not living up to Shapiro's own ideas, goals, and the like. That she criticizes Thompson for not doing in 1933 what she would have been able to do and/or what she is likely to have done in the 1990s is patently distressing. What about mentalizing? Can Thompson rest in peace and still have a mind of her own? Why must Thompson be like Shapiro? This is a most curious way to navigate in the world today as a relational analyst.

> I am not in a position to corroborate or refute Dupont's identification of Clara Thompson as Dm ... but even if Thompson was not abused, the fact that she was a patient and student of Ferenczi during his final years put her in a unique position to spread the word when she returned to America about the reality of abuse and its impact on children's lives. However, she actually did nothing of the sort ...
>
> (Shapiro, 1993, p. 161)

After rereading Sue Shapiro's article (Shapiro, 1993) I find myself thinking about many women who have contributed, worked hard, and made great sacrifices only to be forgotten, maligned, and besmirched. Why do certain people who follow others feel compelled to posthumously take the wind out of their sails? These things I ask myself as I read Sue Shapiro's picking apart of Thompson's character, motivations, ethical behavior and, worst of all, the memories of her patients, whom she intruded upon by interviewing them. It is as if she exhumed Clara Thompson to try her in the court of her patients[2] (Shapiro, 1993).

To be certain, Ferenczi made significant contributions to the field of psychoanalysis in spite of the fact that he had many psychological problems. For one thing, he had various unresolved conflicts that certainly must have influenced the way he worked. He also appeared to be bitter because of Freud's advice about leaving Elma. Who's to say that his resentment and countertransference didn't negatively affect his ability to analyze Clara Thompson?

> From the moment you advised me against Elma, I developed a resistance against your person, that even psychoanalysis could not overcome, and which was responsible for all my sensitivities. With this unconscious grudge in my heart, I followed as a faithful son, all your advice, left Elma, came back to my present wife, and stayed with her in spite of innumerable attempts in other directions.
>
> (Gabbard & Lester, 1994, p. 76)

He also may have identified with Thompson's neediness, which conceivably was off-putting to him, causing him to project those unwanted feelings onto her and, as a result, ridding himself of them. After all, he reportedly never felt loved by his mother (Gabbard & Lester, 1994). Perhaps there was something about Clara Thompson that he couldn't tolerate and that caused him to treat her differently. The "Kissing Technique" with Thompson seemed to be offensive to Ferenczi, yet this was his way of working. "His technique included kissing and hugging the patient like 'an affectionate mother' who 'gives all consideration of one's own convenience, and indulges the patient's wishes and impulses as far as in any way possible'" (Grubrich-Simitis, 1986, p. 272). This of course is only a hypothesis. I can never know what was on Ferenczi's mind when he was analyzing Clara Thompson, but something caused him to feel she was ridiculous and "abandon his hypocritical insensitivity and admit his antipathy and his revulsion …" (Dupont, 1988, pp. 131–132).

With regard to Shapiro (1993) and Brennan (2015), it is of interest to note that the premise on which they built their criticism of Thompson and her parents has been refuted by others. Taylor (2009), a scholar, well-respected MIT senior psychologist and Harvard lecturer, said about Thompson in his book, *The Mystery of Personality: A History of Psychodynamic Theories*:

> Her father was a self-made man … who rose to become president of his own wholesale drug company. Her mother was a quiet but forceful housewife who created a loving household environment [and] who made Clara's early life carefree and untroubled.
>
> (p. 115)

With regard to B. William Brennan (2015), it is obvious that he is a great admirer of Sándor Ferenczi, singing his praises frequently. Unfortunately, he does so at the expense of an important woman in the psychoanalytic field who contributed a great deal beginning in the 1930s.

Brennan begins his article by retelling parts of Shapiro's story (claiming that Thompson, a student and patient of Ferenczi's, was at fault because she told the truth about what happened in her analysis to a fellow candidate). "The incident forever tarnished his [Ferenczi's] reputation …" (Brennan, 2015, p. 78). Brennan added, "The annals of psychoanalytic history are most likely to remember Clara Thompson as the patient who boasted she could kiss Papa Ferenczi whenever she liked" (p. 78). This is curious thinking at best. After all, who is ultimately responsible for the behavior in the consulting room, the analyst or the patient? Who is bound by confidentiality, the analyst or the patient? Can patients tell others what occurs in their treatment? If not, why not? As far as I know, that is not the problem.

Brennan also recounts an interview with Kurt Eissler that Thompson gave for the Freud archive in which she reiterated her assertion: "Sure, I kiss him anytime I want to" (Brennan, 2015, p. 84). I guess telling the story once was not enough for him. He must have had a need to repeat it again for some unknown reason. Without any comment about the imbalance of power inherent in a patient-doctor relationship of this type, Brennan's placing the blame on Thompson is unanalytic to say the very least: The patient, who happens to be a woman, is blamed for the transgressions of the person—a man—who was in charge (or who ought to have been in charge).

The retelling of Shapiro's version of the kissing scenario was questionable enough, but one could say that Brennan was merely reviewing the literature. However, his own speculations about the event are much more damaging.

> It was clearly a mutual enactment, and one in which Thompson replicated the dynamics of childhood boundary crossings and in particular her own confusion between childhood tenderness and adult passion. Ferenczi was enacting his own desire to be a loving mother he never had, since his own mother was unavailable and lacked warmth.
>
> (Brennan, 2015, p. 84)

First of all, as I have noted previously, the word "enactment" was not used in write-ups of this type until 2010 (Aron & Harris, 2010, p. 18). If Brennan had a need to use the word that doesn't really work, then so be it. However, that it was "clearly a mutual enactment" (p. 84) is a risky thing to say, as are the other assertions that he has stated as facts when they are nothing of the sort. They are rumors, untrue statements, debatable renditions of history, or any other word(s) one uses for speculative aspects of the past that have been reported differently by variously sources, e.g., "Thompson replicated the dynamics of childhood boundary crossings," "her own confusion between childhood tenderness and adult passion" (p. 84). These statements are "hypotheses," as is "Ferenczi was enacting his own desire to be a loving mother he never had, since his own mother was unavailable and lacked warmth" (p. 84). How on earth would Brennan know any of these things? And what about Ferenczi's treatment of Elma Laurvik, the daughter of his patient and later wife, Gizella Pálos? Was the same dynamic at play when he debated about whom he should marry after treating both of them (Roazen, 1997)? I wonder why Brennan didn't comment on that situation. If he had done so, it would have helped to create a more balanced picture of Ferenczi's tendency to act inappropriately with female patients versus accusing Thompson of having "forever tarnished Ferenczi's reputation" (Brennan, 2015, p. 78).

With regard to analyzing the motives of people we have never met, is it within our scope of practice to state with such authority what occurred many years before we were born? If anyone thinks that is acceptable, on what basis would that be the case? Of course, I am not talking about putting together facts and forming hypotheses or conducting research and formulating possibilities for the future. I am talking about appearing to know why someone did something in the past based on hearsay, personal notes written in some type of code, making interpretations without knowing or meeting the individual written about. Even if one had process recordings it would be difficult, since it is hard to tell what is happening between two people in a room just by listening to a recording. What about body language and what isn't said? As we all know, it is very risky business to analyze people whom we have never met. If fact, it is against the ethical code of the American Psychiatric Association. One can question what others say, form hypotheses, speculate, but not analyze or say with authority anything about the mental state of another person without examining that person. Putting all that aside, what about the idea of "doing no harm"?

In this current climate of secrecy, projection, projective identification, and alleged false news, perhaps an air of paranoia has entered many people's minds because they are anxious and afraid of what the future holds for all of us. However, in 1993 or 2015 the political atmosphere that has led to so many feelings of confusion and uncertainty did not exist. Why, I wonder, were Shapiro and Brennan so intent on discrediting Clara Thompson?

The kiss-and-tell anecdote is not the only example of Brennan's (2015) possible hostility toward Thompson. Even while chastising her for harmful gossip about Ferenczi, he knowingly presented gossip about her himself: He initially claimed that she had "self-sabotaged" a promising psychiatric residency under Adolf Meyer that "ended abruptly, shrouded in salacious rumors" (Brennan, 2015, p. 78). Pages later he included Thompson's firm written denial that she had been her "analyst's mistress," countering a rumor that Meyer (Brennan, 2015) had apparently believed. "A more sophisticated woman and one less secure in her innocence, would have been more discreet" (p. 83).[3] Brennan (2015) also complained that Thompson was "more critical" (p. 88) of Ferenczi during the final year of his terminal illness with pernicious anemia, when he suffered from mental confusion due to low red-blood-cell counts. He does not attribute Ferenczi's scabrous version of his first encounter with "Dm." (for which there is no evidence) to those same confusions. Instead, he reported Ferenczi's feelings of "disgust" with "Dm." and his struggles "with the fact that she was odoriferous" (p. 90). Brennan (2015) also repeatedly attributes "shame" to Thompson (p. 79), in connection with a supposed lover, among other aspects of her life.[4] Notably, almost all these charges relate to Thompson's sexuality, hence her gender; almost certainly he would not have chastised a man for the same behavior. Certainly he did not make similar comments about Ferenczi's sexuality.

Brennan (2015) concludes that Thompson will probably be remembered only as the person who marred Ferenczi's reputation—even though, by 1993, he had become one of the most admired psychoanalysts in history. There is no doubt that the "kissing" incident occurred, and that Thompson reported it to Jackson (one of Freud's analysands); late in life she referred to it matter-of-factly (another criticism Brennan made about Thompson). Here, a woman has been purged from history as a valuable contributor and made a scapegoat because she did not keep her treatment secret, although the type of treatment, involving sexual relationships with female patients, was her analyst's stock-in-trade at the time.

To turn to my second question about Brennan's attack (Brennan, 2015), which involves the content of Ferenczi's own report, it is evident to any reader of *The Clinical Diary* (Dupont, 1988) that Ferenczi found "Dm." personally and socially repellent. He repeats the comments about her smell, explaining that she perspired "quite conspicuously" and that she had an anal fissure that was apparently problematic for him. "It [becomes] manifest when she suppresses her tendency toward almost manic rage in speech, voice, and gestures" (Dupont, 1988, p. 131). Thompson had a different take on it, however. She thought it was a sexual smell. Ferenczi also reports, from the analytic sessions of "Dm.," that her mother once grabbed her wrist so hard she broke her arm, that she had the odor of a corpse, that she was born with teeth—which Ferenczi interprets as "the strongest [of] aggressive tendencies" (Dupont, 1988, p. 115), that she refused the breast, and that she demanded that he become a "good mother" to her and accept her "tomboy love" before she would "cut loose from her dependence" on him (Dupont, 1988, p. 125). Again, this characterization does not sync up with what Taylor, a well-known Harvard-trained scholar and historian, said (2009). In his book about the contributors of psychoanalytic theory (2009) he indicated her mother provided a "loving family environment that made Clara's early life carefree and untroubled" (Taylor, 2009, p. 115).

Nevertheless, in spite of other renditions of Thompson's life, throughout the chapter in *The Legacy of Sándor Ferenczi: From Ghost to Ancestor* (2015), he seemed to be intent on blaming Thompson for Ferenczi's shortcomings in spite of the fact that few if any of his assertions about Thompson can be corroborated. Apparently, the fact that some of this information is in the diary (Dupont, 1988), it was not enough for Brennan. He had to restate it himself—true or not.

This toxic material, after all, goes far beyond gossip about kissing. It has greatly damaged Clara Thompson's reputation. Why, I wonder, did Brennan stop short of discussing Ferenczi's negative countertransference to "Dm." and how it affected the work? Of course, as indicated earlier, Ferenczi never intended his diary to be published. Yet others decided it was acceptable in spite of the uncertainty of its characterizations and the damage it could do to other people. And, of course, we must remember that Ferenczi's pernicious anemia not only seriously impaired his balance and mobility, but toward the end of his life even brought his thought processes to near-delirium; however, this did not seem to be seriously considered by Brennan, Shapiro or Dupont.

Ferenczi's involvement with a mother and daughter

My final issue with Brennan's view is simple: Freud's critiques of Ferenczi's treatment of women did not begin with the "kissing" episode (Dupont, 1988). As mentioned earlier, Freud was already highly critical of Ferenczi's excessive personal involvement with his patients, so the "kissing" event could only have widened the breach. In addition to the famous December 13 letter in which Freud inserted a reproach to Ferenczi for his pre-analytic tendency for sexual play with patients (Brabant & Falzeder, 2000), as mentioned earlier, Ferenczi also had a complicated triadic relationship with his eventual wife, Gizella Pálos, and her daughter, Elma (15 years his junior), whom he treated and with whom he fell in love during that treatment in 1911[5] (Roazen, 1997). As a psychiatric patient, Elma went back and forth between Ferenczi and Freud (she spent three months with the latter). The two analysts had heated exchanges about Ferenczi's dual relationships: an affair with Gizella before her divorce, and an infatuation with his patient Elma, still of child-bearing age, who was Gizella's daughter.[6] Ferenczi wanted to marry Elma; whether she returned his passion is unclear (Roazen, 1975). Eventually, despite his romantic feelings for Elma, in 1919 Ferenczi decided to marry her mother, Gizella. Unfortunately, through his involvement with her daughter, he had experimented with the psyche of a fragile, depressed young woman in a way that was probably quite traumatic (Roazen, 1997).

This part of Ferenczi's life was apparently a tightly held secret for some time, due in part to the fact that Michael Balint and others admired Ferenczi and did not want his reputation to be damaged (Dupont, 1988). It didn't appear in the literature until the Freud-Ferenczi correspondence came to light in 1994. According to Roazen (1997), the delay occurred because Anna Freud held up the publication for various reasons. No matter what kept the story out of the public eye, to his credit Balint (Roazen, 1997) did write to the young woman who was an unwitting participant in the triangular affair to inquire about her feelings. While he may have participated in the suppression of the story, he at least considered the well-being of Elma Laurvik to some extent by writing a respectful letter to her:

> To write a biography of Sándor ... without mentioning the role you played in his life, would be a falsification, or at least a *suppression veri* [suppression of truth] ... A certain number know (by hearsay) an approximate version of that history, and if the official biograph were to remain silent on this point, it would give rise to fresh gossip and new rumors ... I ask you to think about this very personal and delicate problem.
>
> (Roazen, 1997, para. 24)

However, despite Balint's considerate inquiry, there is a comparison to be made here. Significant damage caused by a male analyst to the life of a 25-year-old patient is quietly hushed up by male colleagues for years. But a young Clara Thompson, who told a fellow student about what was allowed in her analysis, is publicly vilified as having tainted Ferenczi's reputation forever (Roazen, 1997). Should we also blame Thompson for Freud's displeasure over Ferenczi's relations with women patients, which had begun at least 20 years earlier? Must we exonerate and praise one significant contributor who at the same time made life-altering errors, yet denigrate another who devoted her life to the profession, helping many along the way, all because of a personal diary that was not meant to be published, with entries that are sometimes clearly inaccurate?

In light of the fact that Brennan (2015) seemed to present himself as some type of expert on Thompson and Ferenczi, one would certainly assume, at least as a hypothesis, that he knew about Ferenczi's past boundary problems and questionable, as well as inappropriate, behavior with women, some of the same issues that concerned Freud (Brabant & Falzeder, 2000). Given this assumption, why would he rake Clara Thompson over the coals, so to speak, while overlooking the numerous indiscretions of Ferenczi? It is unconscionable that he would sacrifice an important woman in order to glorify Ferenczi. I will not attempt to analyze Brennan's motives, but will say that he did a great deal of damage to the reputation of Clara Thompson for reasons that are not clear. Moreover, I wonder if he would do the same to a man. He certainly didn't in the case of Sándor Ferenczi, but instead put him on a very high pedestal for all to admire. The resurgence of Ferenczi's work was a necessary and vital part of psychoanalytic history; he offered the world a new way of relating to patients. Lewis Aron (2001) has summarized Ferenczi's professional legacy well:

> Ferenczi's work is largely concerned with the heart of the analytic situation, the relationship between patient and analyst. His discoveries were precisely in those areas that are receiving the most lively attention among current psychoanalytic theorists and practitioners. In many respects, in his disagreements with Freud, Ferenczi set the agenda for all the current controversies on the psychoanalytic scene: emphasis on technique versus metapsychology; experience versus insight; subjectivity versus theory; empathy versus interpretation; a two-person psychology versus a one-person psychology.
>
> (p. 162)

Aron (1996), like Stephen Mitchell and Aron (1999), recognized more than two decades ago that Ferenczi is one of our major forefathers who, despite his personal shortcomings, initiated many key inquiries that changed the nature of psychoanalysis. Maintaining their own perspective, Aron (1996) and Mitchell and Aron (1999) also respect Freud's dilemma in coping with Ferenczi's heretical, even subversive techniques for dealing with patients in a deeply personal, empathetic way (Aron & Harris, 2010). Ferenczi's contributions are not eliminated by virtue of stemming in part from his own unresolved transferences, from his genuine need for more analysis, or from his responsiveness to the ideas of his analytic patients. Just as Ferenczi's game-changing ideas must stay in our story of modern psychoanalysis, Clara Thompson's ideas must be reintegrated into our history as well.

Why the suppression of Thompson?

When I first read Brennan's chapter in the book edited by Harris and Kuchuck (2015), I wanted to understand more about his need to criticize and dismiss an early pioneer in our field. Why wouldn't such a careful scholar of text step back and ask himself, "I wonder what motivated Clara Thompson? Am I being fair-minded about the claims I've made?" If he ever considered Thompson's point of view regarding her treatment with Ferenczi, he never let on. It is quite possible that people like Brennan (2015), knowingly or unknowingly, have become aggressors by adding to the hostile treatment of talented women that still exists in our culture, blaming some victims and exonerating at least some perpetrators.

For insight and historical contextualization I turned to a revealing discussion by Nancy Chodorow (1986) on women physicians in leadership roles. Thompson was a female leader in psychoanalytic training, theory, and the psychology of women at a very early time. Chodorow points out that while some women have advanced into leadership in the broad field of psychoanalysis, their routes have been different from those of men. They attain high status because they are good teachers and administrators, with an intuitive ability to help, even nurture, students. For many years women chose not to compete with men for positions at the highly political "top" of institutes and professional associations, because—in the shadow of 19th-century feminism's analysis of "separate spheres"—that was a male world. This choice was especially likely when the women were mothers, and a great many were in that position. This noncompetitive approach went hand in hand with men not wanting women in leadership roles, except perhaps as committee secretaries. All the more remarkable, then, is Thompson's leading two significant institutes before she was 40. To attend to a parallel issue: Although women can be admired, even beloved, as teachers, after a time who remembers the lessons of even a great teacher?

Perhaps most of all, women tended to write less. With publications the primary source of lasting recognition, women have been behind from the start. Thompson was an innovative teacher, an excellent administrator of leading institutions, and author of a useful book and articles.

Regarding another historical point of interest, I have been curious about the whereabouts of Clara Thompson's unpublished papers and letters. When I was the interim director of the Washington School of Psychiatry and director of the Meyer Treatment Center at this same School, I was able to read a few letters that were among the Sullivan papers. I understood at that time that Clara Thompson's unpublished work was at the William Alanson White Institute, as indicated by Sue Shapiro in her article written in 1993: "I also want to thank the William Alanson White Institute for giving me access to Clara Thompson's unpublished papers and letters!" (p. 159).

However, when I inquired about these items, what I learned is that they seemed to have vanished. In a correspondence with one of the former leaders of the Institute, I was told that Clara Thompson's unpublished papers were not there. The individual with whom I corresponded indicated that others had also inquired about Clara Thompson's work. He went on to say that all the inquiries referenced unpublished papers that they believed the White Institute had in its possession, yet this former director who indicated he was the unofficial keeper of the Institute's history knew nothing about them. This is curious, since Shapiro (1993, p. 159) and

Brennan (2015, p. 93) both thanked the Alanson White Institute for allowing them to see the unpublished work of Clara Thompson.

I won't say that the apparent disappearance of Clara Thompson's unpublished papers is a conscious or unconscious projective identification. I don't know that. However, it does seem most unfortunate that unpublished work by a very important person in our psychoanalytic history disappeared or was lost. Again, a tangible example of a lost voice, the voice of a significant contributor to the history of women and the history of psychoanalysis.

All that aside, in spite of Ferenczi's personal problems, I believe he was a brilliant theory-builder and clinician. I think Aron and Harris (1993) summarized this situation very well. Clearly, Ferenczi is one of our forefathers who initiated the interpersonal and relational shift that changed the nature of psychoanalysis. At the same time, Aron and Harris are able to see shortcomings in his work. They also appear to be able to see and respect at least part of Freud's dilemma.

> The refusal in this collection to come to a committed or final conclusion in regard to Ferenczi is deliberate. There is a mystery and difficulty and courageous creativity throughout Ferenczi's life and work. Little is to be gained by perpetuating a myth of villains or heroes … We can admire him, worry about him and question him while seeing him firmly as a crucial figure in our past and a provocative voice in our evolving theory and practice. It is our hope that these papers create more questions than answers and will be seen as elements in a developing dialogue.
>
> *(Aron & Harris, 1993, pp. 39–40)*

Although there is some truth to Freud's analysis of Ferenczi's motives, this should not diminish the value of Ferenczi's discoveries and contributions. It would be easy to trivialize Ferenczi's contributions in his final years by explaining them away as the result of his lingering unresolved negative transference to Freud.

After researching a great deal about Sándor Ferenczi and Clara Thompson, it is clear to me, despite his human foibles, that Ferenczi's ideas contributed greatly to a shift from a largely intellectualized way of being with patients that was of limited use to many to a new way of relating to people with empathy, compassion, and understanding—techniques that have been much more helpful to a large number of patients. At the same time, I do not believe Clara Thompson, the person who is primarily responsible for bringing Ferenczi's thinking to America, has had the recognition she deserves. Thankfully, there are some insightful and scholarly people cited in this chapter who believe in her value as someone who, in addition to contributing many of her own ideas and theories about women, kept Ferenczi's ideas alive. This is in spite of some negative and unfounded claims about her set forth by others: Shapiro (1993) and Brennan (2015). A fair-minded and unbiased assessment of her contributions includes those made by a Swiss psychoanalyst, André Haynal (1997). He said in *Psychoanalysis and Anthropology* that Ferenczi's main successor in America was Clara Thompson mainly because of what she wrote about countertransference and the role of the analyst as well as her general attitude about psychoanalysis.

Paul Roazen, in a new introduction to Clara Thompson's book *Interpersonal Psychoanalysis: The Selected Papers* (2003), succinctly described his sense of her contributions. "…Clara Thompson's position has simply evaporated … the work of Clara Thompson is in a kind of limbo, a no-man's land reserved for people who have seemingly vanished from history" (2003, p. xiii).

Notes

1 See "In The History of the William Alanson White Institute Sixty Years After Thompson" in *Contemporary Psychiatry*, 2017.
2 See note about Sue Shapiro's interviews of Clara Thompson's patients.
3 The estrangement is more likely to have resulted from accusations that Clara Thompson tried to "filter" Meyer's patients to her analyst.
4 Brennan is mistaken about Thompson's "working-class family" (p. 80) that caused her shame (p. 89): Her father was not a pharmacy clerk or pharmacist but, in her adulthood, owner of a drug company; the family was able to educate her at Pembroke (Brown), already an important private university, though not what it would become in the 1960s. Taylor (2009), a highly respected scholar and historian said Thompson's father was the President of his own wholesale drug company. True, in the Depression she needed to make her living in Budapest—she did not have a trust fund—but so would a male professional. The Boston Brahmin Alice Lowell, who Brennan notes (p. 90) scorned Thompson's "lack of education (*Diary*, p. 90)" was a rival analysand. In the early 1930s, "money and background" meant *real* money.
5 The information in the following paragraphs is largely drawn from Paul Roazen, "Elma Laurvik, Ferenczi's Step-Daughter," *JEP* 5, Spring-Fall 1997, unpaginated. Roazen draws on interviews with Michael Balint and the Freud-Ferenczi correspondence, which reveals much.
6 (Gizella was eight years older than Ferenczi.) In love with Elma, Ferenczi asked Freud to ascertain her interest, then to appeal to her mother on his behalf. Freud, evidently against his better judgment, wrote a wordy and convoluted letter to Gizella. When Ferenczi then wrote that the three had decided that Elma should continue her analysis with Freud in Vienna, Freud replied that he has no free hour, but that since "you don't ask about my inclinations and expectations but rather demand of me that I undertake it, then naturally I assent (Letter 264.)" Later Ferenczi confessed he had gone back to Gizella but was now impotent with her.

References

Aron, L. (2001). *A meeting of minds: Mutuality in psychoanalysis*. Mahwah, NJ: Lawrence Erlbaum Associates, Inc.
Aron, L. & Harris, A. (Eds). (1993). *The legacy of Sándor Ferenczi*. London: The Analytic Press.
Aron, L. & Harris, A. (2010). Sándor Ferenczi: Discovery and rediscovery. *Psychoanalytic Perspectives*, 7, 5–42.
Brabant, E. & Falzeder, E. (Eds). (2000). *The correspondence of Sigmund Freud and Sándor Ferenczi Volume 3, 1920–1933*. Cambridge, MA: Harvard University Press.
Brennan, B. W. (2015). Out of the archive/onto the couch. In A. Harris & S. Kuchuck (Eds), *The Legacy of Sándor Ferenczi* (pp. 77–95). New York and London: Routledge.

Chodorow, N. J. (1986). Varieties of leadership among early women psychoanalysts. In L. Dickstein & C. Nadelson (Eds.), *Women physicians in leadership roles* (pp. 45–54). Washington, DC: American Psychiatric Publishing.

Dickens, C. (1861). *Great expectations.* London: Penguin Classics.

Dupont, J. (Ed.). (1988). *The clinical diary of Sándor Ferenczi.* (Michael Balint, Trans.). Cambridge, MA: Harvard University Press.

Gabbard, G. & Lester, E. (1994). *Boundaries and boundary violation in psychoanalysis.* Washington, DC and London: American Psychiatric Publishing, Inc.

Gelles, R. (1993). Family violence. In R. Hampton, T. Gullotta, G. Adams, E. Potter & R. Weissberg (Eds), *Family violence: Prevention and treatment* (pp. 1–24). Newbury Park, CA: SAGE Publications, Inc.

Green, M. F. (Ed) (1964). *Interpersonal psychoanalysis: The selected papers of Clara Thompson.* New York, NY and London: Basic Books.

Harris, A. & Kuchuck, S. (Eds). (2015). *The legacy of Sándor Ferenczi: From ghost to ancestor.* New York, NY and London: Routledge.

Haynal, A. (1997). For a metapsychology of the psychoanalyst: Sándor Ferenczi's quest. *Psychoanalytic Inquiry: A Topical Journal for Mental Health Professionals,* 17(4), 437–458.

Messina, K. E. (2014). Commentary on "transference as a therapeutic instrument": Clara Thompson, a significant but forgotten voice from the past. *Psychiatry: Interpersonal and Biological Processes,* 77(1), 20–24.

Mitchell, S. & Aron, L. (Eds). (1999). *Relational psychoanalysis: The emergence of a tradition.* New York, NY and London: The Analytic Press.

Mitchell, S. A. & Black, M. J. (1995). *Freud and beyond: A history of modern psychoanalytic thought.* New York, NY: Basic Books.

Moulton, R. (1986). Clara Thompson, M.D.: Unassuming leader. In L. Dickstein & C. C. Nadelson (Eds), *Women physicians in leadership roles* (pp. 87–93). Washington, DC: American Psychiatric Publishing.

Roazen, P. (1975). *Freud and his followers.* New York, NY: Alfred A. Knopf.

Roazen, P. (1997). Elma Laurvik, Ferenczi's step-daughter. *JEP, The European Journal of Psychoanalysis,* 5, Spring-Fall.

Shapiro, S. (1993). Clara Thompson: Ferenczi's messenger with half a message. In L. Aron & A. Harris (Eds), *The legacy of Sándor Ferenczi* (pp. 159–174). Hillsdale, NJ: The Analytic Press.

Taylor, E. (2009). *The mystery of personality: A history of psychodynamic theories.* Dordrecht and New York, NY: Springer.

Thompson, C. M. (2003). *Evolution and Development: Psychoanalysis.* New Brunswick, NJ and London: Transaction Publishers.

PART II
Those who have been damaged
Projective identification as a major cause of the erasure

PART II

3
ELEANOR MARX
A little-known activist

Although pushed to the margins in 20th and 21st century political and social history, Eleanor Marx is a woman everyone should know: her efforts resulted in radical changes in our society that are, although transformed, still in place. She helped develop unions in England while participating with the people who laid the groundwork for the Labour Party and the socialist institutions that exist today. She also worked for the advancement of workers and women, giving both causes her fullest attention. Whereas Marx and Engels constructed the theory of communism, according to Rachel Holmes (2014), who wrote about her remarkable yet sad life, Eleanor was the woman who set the tone for social feminism.

Early years

Eleanor Marx was her father's favorite daughter. Nicknamed "Tussy," she seemed full of life from an early age (Holmes, 2014). Of his other children, Marx seemed to think they were *somewhat* like him, whereas Eleanor, he was reported to say, was *just* like him. She also bore a striking physical resemblance to Marx as well as having a similar temperament (Evans, 1998). Marx, a doting father, was the very center of Eleanor's life. As the youngest daughter, she was cosseted not only by him but by her two elder sisters, Jenny and Laura, as well.

"Tussy" was an outgoing child who took responsibility for running the house and acted as a surrogate mother to the other children, which was striking because she was the youngest by ten years. She and her mother were close, confidantes, and she liked to engage her father, by whom she was home-schooled, in a game of chess, often emerging as the victor. According to Holmes (2014), while she was comfortable interacting with children, she spent a great deal of time in the company of grown-ups. Her eyes dark and full of expression, her hair tousled black curls, Eleanor was a fetching child who had always been intelligent, impassioned, and inclined to debate. She had a great fondness for language, literature, music, and theater, but what truly electrified her was radical politics, socialism in particular (Gornick, 2015).

When Eleanor was young, the Marxes lived in near-penury, on essentially no income; they survived on debt, eagerly awaited legacies, constant subsidies from Friedrich Engels, and by pawning household goods. Nevertheless, they strove to keep up middle-class appearances, with a maid and mediocre "young ladies' schools"—in Eleanor's case not until she was ten, since education of girls was not required. The girls' cultural education was enriched from a young age by such free amusements as music at Roman Catholic churches and workingman's concerts at St. Martin's Hall, parental reading aloud—the Brothers Grimm, Homer, Don Quixote, and *The Arabian Nights* (Kapp, 1972).

The girls also memorized and recited Shakespeare. Eleanor learned German at home and also collected stamps. Karl Marx helped Eleanor absorb almost by osmosis his considerable fund of knowledge about philosophy, economics, politics, and the history of workers' oppression, and he shared with her his thoughts about the inevitability of communism. In a nonacademic vein, he taught her about morality and the importance of family. Engels, a friend of the entire Marx family, contributed to Eleanor's education as well. Family entertainment was usually limited to Sunday open houses that, over the years as the Marxes moved from Soho to Kentish Town, drew many people, often European visitors, who debated the politics of the day as well as socialism (Kapp, 1972).

Eleanor was reported to be a happy, outgoing child who spoke up for causes that were important to her. She was always included in discussions about world issues and did not hesitate to offer her opinions in group settings. She was also an avid correspondent, writing her first letter at age six. When she was about nine years old, she even wrote—or dictated—letters to Abraham Lincoln advising about the proper conduct of the Civil War. She also demonstrated leadership skills from an early age. She was undoubtedly what we would call a tomboy (Kapp, 1972).

Holmes (2014) depicted her as having the most extroverted personality of her friends, bringing them home with her, where the housekeeper would treat them to tea and cookies. She was friendly, at ease in most situations, full of laughter, and made all her friends—of whom she was the clear leader—feel welcome and included. So popular was "Tussy" that the entire Marx family came to be known in the neighborhood as "the Tussies."

Growing activism

During Eleanor's early childhood, Marx was working on the first volume of *Das Kapital*. When she got older, she worked with her father, essentially as his personal assistant, which offered her many opportunities that people her age could only dream about. Thereafter, together with Engels, she edited Karl Marx's work. Later she went out into the world and participated actively in what Marx and Engels talked about, work that she edited at the hearth in her family's home (Holmes, 2014).

Her activities also came to include organizing workers to form unions, teaching people in many sectors about socialism as an alternative to capitalism, and advocating for social justice for women. She was brought up as a secularist "free thinker," which led to automatic hostility from Victorian religious believers. Nevertheless, Eleanor had a powerful capacity to understand people. She could put herself in the shoes of others with very different backgrounds from her own family. Early in her activist career, in line with socialist doctrine regarding the education of working people, she proved to be a superb teacher. As a translator and huge admirer of Ibsen, she brought his work—an "impropriety" at the time—to many public places in Britain. She translated Flaubert's *Madame Bovary* into English for the first time. She also taught Shakespeare and Shelley to those who had little exposure to art and culture (Holmes, 2014).

Perhaps Eleanor Marx's deepest commitment lay in helping the working class rise from oppression, a value she had learned from her father and Engels as they explored the ramifications of transforming society. Thus she became one of the initial leaders of the Social Democratic Federation (SDF), the group that evolved from the first socialist organization to focus on workers and working conditions. In 1889 she joined early labor organizer Will Thorne (a gas worker who would become the first general secretary of the Trades Union Congress and eventually a member of Parliament) to launch the National Union of Gas Workers and General Labourers of Great Britain and Ireland. Its platform sought to reduce the working day to eight hours, to establish higher pay rates for Sunday, and more (Holmes, 2014).

Among other achievements for workers, Eleanor served as organizer of various strikes in Britain. She took on many of the less glamorous clerical tasks and participated in marches as well. She co-led the London dock strike, the Silvertown gas-, rubber-, and chemical-workers' strike, and the onion skinners' strike at Crosse & Blackwell, in which she helped 400 women workers get an increase in their salaries, paving the way for Britain's modern labor movement (Holmes, 2014).

After Karl Marx's death in 1883, Eleanor took up more of his tasks as a political organizer. She was a confident orator who could speak in front of very large crowds about issues that were near and dear to her. Unsurprisingly, she was a hard worker, once giving 40 speeches for her causes in a three-month period; one of her most powerful fell on the 15th anniversary of the Paris Commune in 1871, "this first, defeated, proletarian revolution" to which her internationalist's soul was devoted. "When the revolution comes—and it must come—it will be by the workers, without distinction of sex or trade or country, standing and fighting shoulder to shoulder" (Kapp, 1976, p. 82).

In 1886, Eleanor and her partner, Edward Aveling, sailed for New York. While in America Eleanor gave a number of speeches, many about property and production (Holmes, 2014). Before departing she gave a speech in Hyde Park before a crowd of 100,000 people, not an unusual size for her. During that particular rally she was supporting the cause of dockworkers (Kapp, 1976). Upon completion of her tour, Eleanor's view of New York was that it was ideal in terms of location for commerce but hellish because of the inequality that existed (Kapp, 1976). Upon her return to England, she and Aveling wrote *The Working-Class Movement in America*. Her activism was steadfast. She, and for that matter Aveling, always kept in sight their professional goal of emancipating the working class (Holmes, 2014).

"The woman question"

While it was too late for Eleanor, in mid-19th century England, the phrase "the woman question" was used to generalize about a variety of debates over women's place in society. The opposing voices emphasized either the benefit of women having greater educational and political opportunities, or the need for women to remain in the home as caretakers to their families and structural pillars of society. Queen Victoria herself reportedly grappled with the two sides of the woman question since she was at times depicted as the perfect monarch and at other times the good wife (Beard, 2013).

As the middle classes grew with the empire and prosperity, the period even saw an increasing separation of the sexes, with women who did not need to work increasingly represented as, and charged with, creating a home and taking care of children.

Despite this propagandistic appeal, some intelligent women started to insist on more political and legal rights such as owning property and having the ability to become more financially independent. The pioneering figure in the "woman question" had been Mary Wollstonecraft, who in 1792 published *A Vindication of the Rights of Women*, arguing that women were not inferior to men by nature but by lack of a sound education, an opportunity that had for centuries been open only to men. In 1869 Hitchin College—the forerunner of Girton College, Cambridge—was founded, and middle-class young women were permitted to take the London matriculation exams (Kapp, 1972).

Once educated, women and their allies argued, there was no reason why they should not vote, an astonishing claim of near political equality with men. In 1867 (the year in which a reform bill extensively broadened male suffrage) John Stuart Mill founded the London National Society for Women's Suffrage, a male validation for one of the causes that Eleanor Marx would join. For years it failed, even as qualifications for male voters, such as property ownership, were removed one after another and male suffrage became almost universal. The few strides that were made benefited upper-middle-class women; resistance blocked change for most women throughout the century.

But mid-century England also saw the rise of steam engines, railroads and the world's first industrialization, and with it a huge demand for grinding, daylong labor for women as well as men. After all, women could do those repetitive jobs, especially in the thread and cotton mills, and usually more cheaply. The working class emerged and consolidated; women, no longer tied by tradition to home or farm, and needing that extra wage, joined in the throngs heading to the mills, returning at day's end to small, dark, terraced houses to undertake such housework as they had time and energy to do. Given economic need, prostitution seems to have grown as well (Holmes, 2014).

Crucially, Eleanor Marx championed these working-class women more than the bourgeois suffragettes. She was sure that suffrage for middle-class women within existing capitalist society, while necessary, failed to address society's attitude toward working women. Eleanor summarized her view in her own writing on "The Woman Question" (Marx, 1886) in a pamphlet cowritten with her partner. "We must seek the real cause of women's enclaved position in her economic dependence upon man, and ... her 'emancipation' means nothing but economic freedom." According to Eleanor, economic equality was essential if one was to be happy. To be independent, women need to work. A surprisingly modern feminist point of view.

Similar debates were arising in Russia, where the separation of social classes and the rule of the czar were both almost absolute. A few revolutionary writers took up the cause of women's emancipation. One major figure was Nikolai Chernyshevsky, whose 1863 novel *What Is to Be Done?* was written while he was in prison, but became a radical classic across Europe.

It impressed Lenin as well, which must have been music to Eleanor Marx's ears. By the 1890s, many had begun to think that the struggle of the worker and the struggle of the suffragette were the same fight. Eleanor had learned this concept from her father and Engels, who hypothesized that common men could achieve their just place in society only if they fought for equality for women as well. To them, tyranny was tyranny; the proletariat would win only if women and men stood side by side. In fact, Marx, Engels, and Lenin considered oppressed masses of working women the greatest "reserve army" of the proletarian revolution.

After her death, in 1921, V. I. Lenin wrote opinions that furthered her cause. Capitalism, he stated, is doubly injurious to women. Worker or peasant, the woman is crushed by the capitalist. Even in the most democratic of contexts she is unequal to man before the law. Furthermore, in the home women also find themselves in a state of domestic servitude, even slavery, caught up in the drudgery and toil of the kitchen and in their unceasing responsibilities to the family, which they must perform on their own (German, 2010).

Many of the rights, freedoms, and benefits established in modern British democracy—indeed, across Europe—are a direct result of the organizing and advocacy work of Eleanor Marx and women and men like her. She helped to reduce the working day, as well as generally improving safety in workplace conditions. Other common principles of employment that exist today emerged in part through the efforts of these pioneering English socialists: the outlawing of child labor, the formation of unions that ensured workers' ability to bargain collectively and to maintain their rights, and much more challenging, the involvement of women in every aspect of union membership and leadership. At the level of the larger culture, they fought for the rights of everyone, whatever their class or gender, to receive an appropriate education, as well as for universal suffrage. In the long run, their struggles also led to democratically elected parliamentary representation, a thin version of socialism that survives in 2017.

Does projective identification fit the Eleanor Marx story?

Absolutely! In some ways, in fact, it *is* the story; a better example would be hard to find. In 1898, Eleanor died of cyanide poisoning, without question. Some say she committed suicide because she was depressed, but other accounts indicate that she was not feeling suicidal at the time of her death or during that period of her life. Many have speculated that the cause of her death was murder, and, spurred by statements sympathetic to Eleanor, socialist newspapers at the time explored the matter in lurid detail (Holmes, 2014).

In the early 1880s Eleanor had fallen in love with a married man. When she was 27 years old, Eleanor met Edward Aveling—freethinker, biology teacher, disciple of Darwin—in the British Museum's reading room. He was a fellow atheist, a theatrical man in every sense, and a well-trained scientist. By early December of 1883 they had become lovers (an unconventional if not scandalous matter, except that socialism sanctioned radical-style "free love"), and starting in 1884 they lived in a common-law arrangement for 14 years. Initially, Eleanor seemed to have gained confidence and authority from their partnership: she began to appear in public much more. Other people, however, thought he was a cad (Hughes, 2014).

Throughout their years together, Eleanor continued her organizing efforts and public advocacy. During that time they were together, she drew him into her innermost political circles. Soon they were a power couple, with Aveling on the podium as often as Eleanor. It was her extraordinary energy that almost invariably led the intellectual way, but they were a remarkably successful team; her intellectual passion, her political high-mindedness, her steadfast devotion to the cause—for all this he loved her. Yet he told her that he couldn't marry her because he was already married and lied that he couldn't get a divorce. Unfortunately for Eleanor, Edward later concealed the fact of his wife's death. He reportedly hungered for good clothes, expensive restaurants, cabs, and theater tickets, and was indifferent as to how those desires were satisfied. The person at whose expense Aveling generally made himself comfortable was, of course, Eleanor.

According to Gornick (2015), Aveling was selfish, nasty, petty, and three times out of five not there when Eleanor needed him. A hypochondriac of some dimension, he was forever going off to take "the cure" somewhere (really to rendezvous with other women), leaving Eleanor alone for weeks on end. As the years went on, the discrepancy between a crowded public life and a lonely personal one weighed ever more heavily on her.

The singular Aveling was, from a moral perspective, something of an "optical illusion": Viewed from one angle he was a man of few cares with an essentially sound composition; viewed from another he was thoroughly and indisputably disreputable. What was plain to all, however, was his parasitic bent, a chronic tendency to borrow money from anyone, rich or poor, at times to their financial ruin (Kapp, 1976).

Disasters began to pile up. In August 1895 Eleanor's dear "second father," Friedrich Engels, died. In the same month Eleanor learned that Freddy Demuth, a close friend for a decade, was not in fact Engels's illegitimate son but Karl Marx's son by a beloved housekeeper—and fostered out, then ignored by their father. Eleanor began to spiral downward as Aveling's lies continued. Although she was unaware of his latest deception; in June 1897, under an alias, Edward secretly married 22-year-old Eva Frye, a young actress, and two months later left the home he had shared with Eleanor.

In a few days he returned, probably after consulting counsel about his financial position. Eleanor took him back and spent six bitter months nursing her partner's recurrent, and ultimately fatal, kidney disease. Eventually it became apparent even to Eleanor that Aveling stayed with her only for medical and financial support. She was forced to confront some of his lies and deception, including the fact that he had hoped to inherit his first wife's money, and that he now sought Eleanor's estate, including what Engels had willed to her, and control of Marx's *Nachlass*, or literary estate (Kapp, 1976).

Eleanor learned that Aveling had remarried, sometime between Sunday, March 27 and Thursday, March 31 (Holmes, 2014). Just prior to that time, finally realizing more and more about Aveling's deceptive ways, she tried to change her will, probably removing Aveling as her primary beneficiary, but her final codicil did not reach her solicitor (Kapp, 1976).

After taking advantage of Eleanor for years, Aveling finally discharged the destructive force that was aimed at her for so long; he blew up the very foundation of her life when she was only 43. If he didn't cause her death directly, he certainly could easily have prevented it. He should have known what was likely to happen on that desperate day in March 1898. With regard to the prussic acid that she ingested, his initials were on the note to the pharmacist (Kapp, 1976). One way or the other, directly or indirectly, he had already spewed the toxic content of his disdain and contempt toward his victim until it killed her, either literally or as a metaphor for her bruised heart. Whether by manslaughter or suicide, Edward Aveling played the part of the abuser who caused Eleanor Marx's death. He also did not claim her ashes (Holmes, 2014). He did, however, inherit her estate. Aveling was granted probate, then ran through 1,000 pounds—perhaps paying a debt or two, a bribe or two—in the 16 weeks before his own death (Kapp, 1976).

Eleanor's too-little-known contributions to democracy and social justice were lost in part because the concept of a woman socialist activist could barely be acknowledged in early studies of socialist/communist history. Another reason her contributions were suppressed in Victorian England, no doubt, is the disgrace of her unconventional relationship, its humiliating end, and her possible, perhaps "guilty" suicide. Nevertheless, Eleanor Marx's legacy is alive and well in the minds of many British people. Her relationship with Aveling is also an excellent example of projective identification. It can initially start when women are projected upon without fully understanding what has occurred, knowing something is off but not really wanting to know the truth. Eleanor wanted to believe Aveling until the evidence became too clear. By then it was too late, either because he killed her or because she was overcome with a sense of despair.

Generally speaking, dilemmas of this type continue until the dynamics shift. In "giving back projections," so to speak, one must confront his or her betrayer. Only in this way can wrongs be righted, only in this way is repair possible, and only in this way can offenders begin to learn the process of mentalizing or how to function in a two-minds process (more about this topic will be discussed in Chapters 13 and 14).

References

Beard, J. (2013, January 9). Yes, she was stroppy, but Queen Victoria dearly loved her children. *The Guardian*.

Chernyshevsky, N. (1986). *What is to be done?* (N. Dole and S. S. Skidelsky, Trans.). Ann Arbor, MI: Ardis.

Evans, F. (1998, April 1). Eleanor Marx was fearless in her pursuit of bohemian ideals, but ultimately constrained by her traditional roles as daughter and lover. *The Independent*.

German, A. B. (2010). *The great Soviet encyclopedia* (3rd ed., 1970–1979). (Vol. 42), pp. 368–369. Moscow: Soviet Encyclopedia Publishing House.

Gornick, V. (2015, April 3). The life of a daughter of the revolution. *International New York Times*.

Holmes, R. (2014). *Eleanor Marx*. London: Bloomsbury Publishing Co.

Hughes, K. (2014, May 16). Review of Rachel Holmes, Eleanor Marx: A life. *The Guardian*.

Kapp, Y. (1972, 1976). *Eleanor Marx*. (Vols. 1–2). New York, NY: Pantheon Books.

Marx, E. (1886). The woman question: From a socialist point of view. *Westminster Review*, No. 125, London, January–April (first printed as a separate stand-alone edition by Swan Sonnenschein & Co. London, 1986).

Wollstonecraft, M. (1996). *Mary Wollstonecraft: The vindication of the rights of women*. Mineola, NY and New York, NY: Dover Publications, Inc.

4

A 21ST CENTURY WOMAN

Anne Case

I became interested in reading articles about Anne Case because she seemed to be one of the women who was working successfully in what had been a "man's world." She seemed like someone who had profited from the second wave of feminism that began in the 1960s. Case has a Ph.D. and has held the Alexander Stewart Chair in Economics and Public Affairs at Princeton University. She has also worked side by side with her husband, Angus Deaton, Ph.D., for three decades. They traveled to developing countries around the world conducting research to determine the relationship among mortality rates, inequality, and poverty, work they began long before inequality began to be seen as one of society's most pressing problems.

In the winter and spring of 2016–17, Case and Deaton's studies of rising mortality rates among middle-class white Americans, utilizing more than 15 years of data, received a blizzard of media publicity following their September 2016 article in *Proceedings of the National Academy of Sciences*. Like all academic research, this study has its critics and detractors. In one blog, for instance, Andrew Gelman (2017) questioned the Case and Deaton story by pointing to its sensationalistic coverage, including the lack of scholarly critique from other disciplines.

When the original Case-Deaton story came out, questions were raised about the methodology. Critics asked why the data were not filtered by educational level or by state, which are research questions available for other scholars to pursue. Other detractors have pointed out that, even if the morbidity and mortality of African-Americans did not increase in the period studied, they still had higher death rates than those of white people; thus, the Case and Deaton report could permit those who wish to turn their backs on the black plight to do so. Recently, Case and Deaton came under fire for their work in this area (Gelman, 2017). None of these criticisms, however, fault the authors' results or interpretation per se.

It was business as usual at this point. The media listed this major study's authors as "Case and Deaton"—the woman first, which would be expected since the order of authors of journal articles in economics is listed based on the level of participation of the researchers. The "senior" or "lead" author, who usually designed the study, appears first. For many years in their work together, professors Deaton and Case have distinguished which of the two is the senior author, and they did so for the *PNAS* study.

So, all was well as I perused the news of world events. Then one day I saw an article in *The New York Times* that referred to the Nobel Prize in Economics and something that had been said by David Plotz in a political pod-cast (Wolfers, 2015). What caught my eye was the title: Nobel Prize-winning economist Angus Deaton and Anne Case, who is his wife, and also a researcher.

The use of the word "wife," along with the phrase "and also a researcher" seemed to exhibit a subtle gender bias that I was not used to encountering when reading about Case and Deaton. Consciously or unconsciously, the reporter seemed to be describing an event the way it would have been described many years ago, i.e., the man wins a prize and the dutiful wife stands by his side in support of his accomplishments. This would have been acceptable if it were describing the situation accurately, but that wasn't the case. I read on.

In this article in *The New York Times*, "Even Famous Female Economists Get No Respect" (2015), Justin Wolfers said that frequently women still get the short end of the stick. Wolfers (2015) elaborates by describing a paper written by Adam Davidson that gives full credentials to Lawrence Katz—a Harvard professor and scholar of education economics—and mentions the coauthor, Claudia Goldin, by name only. The article fails to mention that Goldin was also a Harvard professor and scholar of education economics, among other things, and perhaps most important, omits the fact that she was actually the paper's first author.

As it turns out, the more I read, the more I realized that journalists, except for a very few financial writers, seem to believe that a woman economist is something akin to a unicorn. The Goldin instance represents intellectual damage that may seem mild to those whose careers are not at stake; for those whose careers are on the line, however, it's a serious matter.

Then I read that Ralph Nader (Wolfers, 2015) decided to enter the debate on monetary policy with an open letter to Janet Yellen, the Chair of the Board of Governors of the Federal Reserve Bank. It was, to be charitable, a rather confused missive—and confusing enough that we might see Mr. Nader as a more successful presidential candidate than economist. But the real flub came with his advice to Ms. Yellen indicating that he thought she should have a talk with her husband, who had won the Nobel Prize, so together they could figure out the right course of action. This is embarrassing evidence of condescension to the most influential woman economist in America.

Wolfers (2015) begins to address the many issues that women in economics face today: why, he asks, would Janet Yellen need her husband's assistance in this matter when she could be considered the world's preeminent economist? Why, with hundreds of Ph.D. economists in her employ, would she require her husband's assistance in the first place? What's more, Wolfers continues, while Mr. Akerlof may be a "brilliant" economic theorist, the man certainly would not claim to be an authority on monetary policy.

In spite of the fact that Mr. Wolfers is obviously trying, his "defense" of Janet Yellen is a bit patronizing. "In her own right" hints at second-class citizenship in the world of economics where Professor Akerlof holds the initial "right," and her potential need for that army of economists at the Fed to help her feminine intellect is not much better. Many years ago, she turned her attention from technical economics to public policy, with a special interest in unemployment, in which she is inarguably more of an expert than Akerlof. When President Barack Obama appointed Yellen to the chairmanship of the Fed, she had previously served as vice-chair under the deeply respected Ben Bernanke. She is almost universally considered successful for leading the management of monetary policy that cut unemployment, kept inflation minimal, and began to wind down the Fed's support of the American economy during the 2008–10 recession.

In a break with bipartisan tradition, President Donald Trump declined to reappoint her to a second term, which is "stunningly unusual," according to Peter Conti-Brown (cited in Van Dam, 2017), financial historian at Penn's Wharton School, of which Trump is a very proud alumnus. Her male replacement has far less preparation than she and no announced policy differences. This pointless gesture of change may be just one more of Trump's moves to obliterate Obama's record. But it may have a more sexist meaning: among Yellen's less-quantifiable practices at the Fed were her ability to listen, to bridge differences among divided governors, and to attend to the human impact of macroeconomic policy (Van Dam, 2017).

Yellen and Akerlof are, to be sure, happily married. In an interview with Mervyn King (Yellen's counterpart as retired chair of the Bank of England), on the day after announcing her plan to depart from the Fed she said, referring to their dinner table, that they discuss more economics than others might find appealing, adding that they even talk about the topic at the beach (Appelbaum, 2017).

Women economists and the academy

Success in modern economics requires not only a high order of mathematical and statistical talent but the ability to pose questions in ways that produce verifiable evidence. Robust results may be questioned by alternative arguments and interpretations, but not decried as mere anecdote. Thus, economists consider themselves the "hardest" of the social and behavioral scientists, with a rigor parallel to that of physics and chemistry. This attitude permeates the field of economics and keeps it a male-dominated profession.

Romero (2013) consulted the National Science Foundation's Survey of Earned Doctorates and found that, in 2011, 34 percent of Ph.D.s in economics were earned by women, which, although it sounds impressive, pales in comparison to the percentage of doctoral degrees earned by women (46 percent), and comprises the smallest portion of any of the social sciences. In psychology, Romero points out, women earned 72 percent of Ph.D.s, while in sociology the percentage of woman-earned Ph.D.s was 61. In economics, says Romero, a phenomenon called the "leaky pipeline" is in effect: at each stage of the profession the gender gap increases. In 2012, according to the Committee on the Status of Women in the Economics Profession (CSWEP), the figures were as such for women: assistant professor (28 percent), associate professor with tenure (22 percent), full professor (less than 12 percent). Possibly these figures are a reflection of the "time lag" between earning a Ph.D. and becoming full professor: if a greater number of women are going into economics today than two decades ago, more women might become full professors a few years down the line. But the percentage of new female Ph.D. students in economics has actually dropped since 1997, when CSWEP first began to collect data.

One example of a woman in this category is Katharine Coman. A graduate of the University of Michigan and already a full professor of history and economics at Wellesley College, she was the only woman at the 1885 meeting at which the American Economic Association was formed. In 1911, Coman published the first article in the inaugural issue of the Association's flagship journal, the *American Economic Review*, assessing the still-critical topic of irrigation in the American West. Whatever her male colleagues thought of Wellesley (where she offered the first course in political economy), they had to grudgingly acknowledge her mentors at Michigan, a major site for the American adaptation of inductive study of economic institutions that had been pioneered by the prestigious German school. After Coman no memorable women appear in the academy until (and except) British post-Keynesian economic theorist Joan Robinson (1903–83) (Madden, 2002). There seems to have been a tacit agreement in the field that women may be given only bit parts, or left off the playbill altogether.

Why did male economists pay so little attention to the women in their midst? Madden (2002) explained by summarizing previous research into women's publications and doctoral dissertations in the early years in "a quantitative report of the frequency of publication, degree status, publication outlets, and the subject matter addressed" by more than 1,000 women in North America and Europe. She takes as a methodological question "Why economists are generally unaware of the contributions of women ... in the early decades of the twentieth century" (p. 3). She demonstrated that women published in all kinds of outlets, including the *Economics Journal* and the *AER*, but also agricultural, labor, history, business, statistical, sociology, and political science journals, as well as government documents and public-interest magazines like *The New Statesman* (Madden, 2002).

Madden's (2002) key finding was that, although men and women published on similar topics, men dominated fields like economic theory and money, credit, and banking—the core of the discipline in the Keynesian and neoclassical, market-based eras—while women wrote about labor markets, productivity, and wages; industry-specific studies; public labor policy and wage policy; legislation, regulation, and economic justice; consumer economics; cost of living and living standards; children; and public responses to poverty.

Many of these subject categories were until recently stereotypically "female-centric," and therefore marginalized in the profession: the *AER* scheme as of 2002 did not include the economics of gender; children, race, and religion; or the economics of the domestic sector. Moreover, according to Madden (2002), for the first half of the 20th century women's contributions tended to be in the areas of data and statistics, with very little mathematical theory. She concludes that women have been inaccurately characterized as outsiders. Stereotyping the economic work of women, she says, is both unfair and inaccurate.

Many years later, do the research topics that have most interested Anne Case, including economic development, still risk this pigeonhole? Like most academic disciplines, economics does not produce rafts of celebrities or *New York Times* best-selling authors. Those who reach public attention, male or female, are likely to have chosen as one field of specialty public policy and to have risen to important positions in civil society, public affairs, or finance. By definition they have stepped outside academia for long periods. Among women, those who have taken those steps include:

- the late Juanita Kreps, secretary of commerce under Jimmy Carter and scholar of labor demographics;
- Isabel Sawhill, fellow and former vice-president of the Brookings Institution, associate director of OMB under Bill Clinton, and informed advocate for delayed childbearing;
- Martina von Neumann Whitman, professor at the University of Michigan's Gerald R. Ford School of Public Policy and Ross School of Business, former vice-president of General Motors and member of the President's Council of Economic Advisors under Richard Nixon;
- Alice Rivlin, founding director of the Congressional Budget Office, director of OMB and vice-chair of the Federal Reserve Board of Governors under Bill Clinton, and expert in fiscal management and debt reduction;
- Abby Joseph Cohen, former chief investment officer and leader of the Global Markets Institute at Goldman Sachs and "bullish" financial analyst;
- Laura D'Andrea Tyson, professor at the Haas School of Business at U.C. Berkeley, chair of the President's Council of Economic Advisers under Bill Clinton, and scholar of trade and international competitiveness;
- Christina D. Romer, Garff B. Wilson Professor of Economics at U.C. Berkeley, chair of the President's Council of Economic Advisers under Barack Obama, coauthor of the administration's plan for recovery from the 2008 recession;
- more recently Heidi Hartmann, founding director of the Institute for Women's Policy and Research and expert on women's employment, women, and Social Security, and the wage gap;

- Caroline Hoxby, chaired professor of economics at Stanford and scholar of higher-education policy, especially college costs and expanding access.

Many of these women were initially educated at Smith, Wellesley, Bryn Mawr, and the like, where men did not outnumber them; several have well-known fathers or husbands, whom journalists and biographers invariably cite. Although most were too busy in their civic careers to produce the intensive research and publication that wins academic prizes, they demonstrate the power of women economists and the social value of economic expertise.

As the presence of women on college and university economics faculties gradually grows, making female students more likely to see role models who look like them and might inspire them, are more young women entering the "pipeline" that might lead them to a Ph.D. and/or professional career? In a working paper in 2010, education economist Claudia Goldin of Harvard, using a highly selective Eastern liberal arts college as her model, asked why young women do not choose economics as a major at the same rate as men and spoke of the large differences, differences that are remaining constant. At Goldin's specimen college, 19.5 percent of men major in economics as compared to about 10 percent for women, a two-to-one ratio that is comparable to peer institutions. When considering course enrollments, Goldin discovered that women dropped out of the required four-course introductory sequence at a greater rate than men, especially if their grades were not A or A-, whereas males' grades did not deter them, apparently because they had greater confidence in their career goals. Sure enough, at graduation the remaining women economics majors have higher GPAs than men (Goldin, 2010). After excluding general math ability and the AP economics exams as significant causes for the marked gender difference, Goldin has no choice but to speculate.

Case and Deaton, women, and the Nobel Prize

Professor Deaton ("Sir Angus" as of December 2016) was professor of economics and international affairs emeritus at Princeton, and senior scholar at the Woodrow Wilson School. Deaton won the Nobel Memorial Prize in Economic Sciences in 2015 for his analysis of consumption, poverty, in his book *The Great Escape: Health, Wealth, and the Origins of Inequality* (Deaton, 2013). Case was not so honored. Her absence from the stage occurred despite the fact that her work, both with Deaton and on her own, laid some of the groundwork for Deaton's accomplishment. While their independent research is far from identical in terms of site, hypothesis, or data sets—and Deaton's scope is notably more historical and econometric—their work was similar in terms of the topics and methods they undertake, yet Case was not mentioned by the Nobel Prize Committee (Wearden, 2015).

If Deaton (2013) had included Case by more extensive reference in *The Great Escape*, would the Nobel Prize Committee have been more likely to include her as a prizewinner? Is her professional training not equal to his? Is her research not similarly innovative? Did she not publish as many articles at a similar career stage? I would like to tease out potential reasons why the Nobel Prize Committee might have treated Anne Case differently. Beyond the journalistic and academic bias, I have already demonstrated, is anything else at play?

The extraordinary and original grasp of history and economic theory in *The Great Escape* was not a thesis Deaton arrived at in 2013 or shortly before; rather, it drew upon information accrued from work with others for many years. Deaton won the Nobel because of what came before his book: the whole picture. He emphasizes this concept in his book when discussing well-being. Surely it must apply to his major hypotheses: "[It] cannot be judged ... without looking at the whole" (Deaton, 2013, p. 9). Deaton's work with Case, with whom he uncovered so much over the years, is an example of the crucial nature of "the whole." Deaton frequently acknowledges Case with helping to edit both his papers and *The Great Escape*, but what about her contributions to his work? He often alludes to concepts they worked on together. For example, in *The Great Escape* (Deaton, 2013) he makes the unsurprising claim that it is very important to study health when talking about societal well-being, and health had been a part of his work for at least a decade. Meanwhile, in "Stature and Status: Height, Ability and Labor Market Outcomes," published in 2006 by the National Bureau of Economic Research, Case and Christina Paxson presented a surprising finding: Children from advantaged backgrounds (what we often call "privilege," including better diet and health care) are likelier to have earlier growth spurts, grow taller, develop more cognitive ability—and earn more money in their adult lives. The relation of health to equality is obvious here, yet Deaton (2013) does not cite Case and Paxson's (2008) important paper, in spite of its apparent relevance. Other examples of Case's work, although not as comparative or historical as Deaton's book, lie in similar fields of investigation to his subject and provide new knowledge. Scholarly teams make decisions on citations as they wish. Would Case's inclusion in Deaton's book have made her look more like a research assistant?

Anne Case and her generation of women

Anne Catherine Case belongs to the generation of women that has followed Janet Yellen. She graduated first in her class from the State University of New York at Albany in 1980 and earned her Ph.D. from Princeton in 1988. She taught at Harvard before becoming assistant professor of economics and public affairs in Princeton's Woodrow Wilson School of Public and International Affairs in 1991; she rose through the ranks from there. Through 2017 Case published 62 articles and book chapters, 52 of them coauthored, nine with Deaton. Clearly, she is generous with credit, and her coauthors are overwhelmingly women, including her most frequent colleague, Paxson. Her publication record demonstrates both her close collaboration with Deaton on such issues as health, aging, and morbidity related to work and gender, in South Africa and India as well as the United States, but also, importantly, the independent research agenda around children that marks her as her own woman. Case has also circulated numerous working papers for discussion, a collegial norm for economists.

In terms of national and international recognition, she has won a dozen fellowships, scholarships, and awards, including from the Econometrics Society and the International Health Economics Society; she has been elected to the American Academy of Arts and Sciences, the American Philosophical Society, and the National Academy of Medicine. In service to her profession, Case has fulfilled time-consuming editorships at *The American Economic Review, Journal of Development Economics, The World Bank Economic Review, The Economic Journal, Journal of Economic Literature*, and *Journal of Economic Perspectives*.

At Princeton she was director of the research program in development studies. Nationally she serves on the NIH National Research Advisory Council on Child Health and Human Development and on the President's Committee for the National Medal of Science, markers of her high stature in the world of biological and medical sciences. This record of academic accomplishment and service is simply stellar. But nobody can be said unequivocally to "deserve" the Nobel Prize.

I wondered how, aside from its much-discussed political emphases in some fields, the Nobel Prize Committee, a private nonprofit organization that works in complete secrecy, selects winners each year. Judging by results, its members have a preconception, perhaps unconscious, that women are less deserving than men of the world's most prestigious award for rigorous thinking and originally designed research. The prizes for literature and peace, which reward imagination, verbal brilliance, and social action? Women have a fair chance, at least in recent years. Of course, the committee members, many of them not young, may be burdened with the negative influences of prejudice that are part of Western cultural "knowledge" about women, subconscious thoughts that are not accessible to us on demand. Study after study has revealed that cultural preconceptions about women as less capable in science, mathematics, engineering, and technology pervade all levels of the career ladder; the Nobel, at the very top, is just the most powerful. Thus, the committee members, even though they hail from progressive Sweden, may fall prey to the same deep sense of gender disparity with which many consciously struggle, because familial and cultural influences are hard to overcome. After all, in 1903 the committee of that era awarded the prize in physics to Pierre and Marie Curie, apparently convinced that a man must have led the key discovery, assisted by the woman involved, an utterly mistaken conviction (Long, 2012). To add insult to injury, Curie actually was slated to win a second Nobel Prize but was asked not to attend the ceremony because there was a scandal about her having an affair with a married man five years after her husband died. Now I ask, would this ever have happened to a man (Krulwich, 2010)?

The final committee cannot solely be blamed for the results of an entire process. For one thing, an awardee has to be nominated by a select group of people: members of the Nobel board of directors, cabinet members, judges from The Hague or members of the Institut de Droit, former awardees, former advisors to the selection committee. University professors can nominate people as well, but they must be drawn from the following departments only: history, social science, law, philosophy, theology, religion. Yet the categories for which achievement is awarded are physics, chemistry, literature, peace, and physiology or medicine (economics was a later addition, established in honor of Alfred Nobel by Sveriges Riksbank, Swedish National Bank). It is true that, when Nobel established the prizes in 1901, different disciplines were admired than those that rank highly today, and the sciences were not so prominent. When all is said and done, however, nominators often cannot name those in their own fields of expertise, while knowledgeable people in the prizewinning fields are not eligible to nominate. Within both groups of disciplines there are subtle and not-so-subtle suggestions that women and their work may be little respected, little known, or little wanted. There is a cultural bias and more: it is not known how men who do support them really feel (Rice, 2011).

I must note that the Nobel committee is very aware of the underrepresentation of women, at least in the early years. As of spring 2017, the home page of its website was headlined "Women Who Changed the World"; it featured headshots of the 49 women who have won Nobel Prizes from 1901 through 2017 (out of a total of 923 prizewinners, which amounts to 18.84 percent); 19 have won since 2001 (Kirk, 2015). Of the 79 individuals who have taken the prize in economic sciences since 1969, one woman is a winner: Elinor Ostrom, who was awarded the prize in 2009.

Can women's achievements in economics—and perhaps, by analogy, in other "hard" academic disciplines—be better recognized? The discipline, represented by its male adherents, seems clearly to have practiced a professional form of projective identification by failing to "give credit where credit is due" to women, whose historical role in developing the discipline (in fields like agricultural economics, employment economics, and, yes, home economics) has been treated as an embarrassment until very recently. The field has allowed some of its accepted subdisciplines to be perceived as "softer" (with feminine overtones) because they have too many unmeasurable variables to permit robust results, and other invented justifications. Economics has valorized abstruse theory rather than practical situations in which economic knowledge and thought might make major differences in human lives—until Janet Yellen came along and quietly demanded a different focus. The cultural atmosphere of a men's club, hinted at in journalists' reports, has been all too comfortable. Until quite recently, that has been true not only in academia but in Washington policy circles, where the field is a profession rather than a discipline: women were not welcomed in the front door (and still are not as welcomed as men).

According to Mundy (2015), just 44 women have served in the Unites States Senate since its inception. She describes the atmosphere in the chamber as one of sexism on every scale. In the 20th century, male senators were inclined to behave like frat boys whose alcohol-stoked state contributed to their predatory sexual activities with subordinate women of all descriptions. Today's female senators, she says, face an undermining, subtler form of sexism and are made to feel that they do not quite belong, which many are loath to admit in the face of the glacial progress that has been made.

Of what are the male resisters in politics, economics, or any other field or profession trying to rid themselves by their unwelcoming stance to women colleagues? For some, fear that they too might be committing professional sins, even in the valorized subdisciplines, by producing tiny and sterile results. For others, conscious or unconscious awareness that the woman in the office next door may be more talented and productive than they, but paid less and promoted less rapidly. How can male economists take back the negativity they have spewed? Treat women economists as individuals independent of their husbands. Look for, appoint to good positions, and reward innovative talent in every subdiscipline of the field, regardless of its "applied" character —or the gender of the economist. And nominate women for the glittering prizes.

There is some good news, though, in economics! At the beginning of last year, the annual meeting of the American Economic Association for 2017–18 made the front page of *The New York Times* (January 11, 2018) and the *PBS News Hour* with a startling new feature: a panel stocked with women economists. Each presented her research on gender bias in the profession, citing virtually all the barriers to progress that I have sketched.

In order to have their writing accepted by prominent economic journals, women must be clearer writers than men (by six percent), says Erin Hengel, an economist at the University of Liverpool. Women wait longer for their work to appear in journals, and in the most popular economics textbooks, men are referred to four times as often as women. The panel learned from Betsey Stevenson, an economist from the University of Michigan, that women depicted in textbook examples are more apt to be shopping or cleaning than creating public policy or heading up a company. More than half of those references concerned Janet L. Yellen. Two prominent female academicians, Janet Currie and Claudia Goldin, both Ivy League economists, discovered that when women cowrite papers with men they tend to get significantly less credit than their coauthors; this is borne out in how the paper affects their likelihood of receiving tenure (Tankersley & Scheiber, 2018). But in 2017 a new twist came to the attention of *The Times*' reporters: a paper by Alice Wu about a widely read anonymous website called Economics Job Market Rumors with a message board that harasses women with crude, sexualized terms (Eisner, 2017).

Essentially, is seems like projection is everywhere. This time the AEA decided to take action, perhaps noticing that progress in women's advancement in economics had stagnated since 2006 and that women's entry into economics was now behind that of the STEM fields. They set up a new, presumably secure online job site and to draft a code of ethical conduct for economists (Eisner, 2017). Were they responding to the quantitative evidence that the women's panel laid before them? If they had consulted their own Commission on the Status of Women in the Economics Profession, they would have discovered that such evidence has been around for a long time.

References

Appelbaum, B. (2017, November 21). As her last day with the Fed nears, Janet Yellen looks back on her first. *The New York Times.*
Case, A. & Paxson, C. (2006). *Stature and status: Height, ability, and labor market outcomes.* National Bureau of Economic Research Working Paper 12466.
Case, A. & Paxson, C. (2008). Stature and status: Height, ability, and labor market outcomes. *Journal of Political Economy, 116*(3), 499–532.
Deaton, A. (2013). *The great escape: Health, wealth, and the origins of inequality.* Princeton, NJ: Princeton University Press.
Eisner, E. (2017). UC Berkeley Blog, Economics.
Gelman, A. (2017, March 24). No-op: The case of Case and Deaton. Andrewgelman.com.
Goldin, C. (2010). Gender and the undergraduate economics major (Unpublished discussion paper). Harvard University.
Kirk, A. (2015, October 12). Nobel Prize winners: How many women have won awards? *The Telegraph.*
Krulwich, R. (2010). Don't come to Stockholm! Madame Curie's Nobel scandal. NPR. Retrieved from www.npr.org/sections/krulwich/2010/12/14/132031977/don-t-come-to-stockholm-madame-curie-s-nobel-scandal.
Long, T. (2012). Jan. 23, 1911: Science academy tells Madame Curie, *"non."* Wired.
Madden, K. K. (2002). Female contributions to economic thought, 1900–1940. *History of Political Economy, 34*(1), 1–30.
Mundy, L. (2015, January/February). The secret history of women in the Senate. *Politico Magazine.*
Nobel Prizes and Laureates. (2009). The Sveriges Riksbank Prize in economic sciences in memory of Alfred Nobel 2009. Nobelprize.org.
Rice, C. (2011). The Nobel Peace Prize's problem with women. Curt-rice.com.
Romero, J. (2013). Where are the women? *Econ Focus*, Second Quarter. Richmondfed.org.
Tankersley, J. & Scheiber, N. (2018, January 10). Wielding data, women force a reckoning over bias in the economics field. *The New York Times.*
Van Dam, A. (2017, December 12). Janet Yellen is on the way out. Trump can totally remake the Fed. Here's why. *The Washington Post.*
Wearden, G. (2015, October 12). Nobel prize in economics won by Angus Deaton—As it happened. *The Guardian.*
Wolfers, J. (2015, November 11). Even famous female economists get no respect. *The New York Times.*

5
HILLARY CLINTON AND THE 2016 PRESIDENTIAL ELECTION

Hillary Clinton did not, of course, "lose" the presidential election of 2016. Thanks to nearly three million more votes than Donald Trump, she won the popular vote. Nevertheless, on November 9 she was not the president-elect because the United States uses the Electoral College, enshrined in our Constitution, which may or may not reflect what the majority of citizens of the country want.[1] No matter how brilliant the Founders were, what they said and wrote is 230 years old and visibly dated. The structure they devised for apportioning representation in the House of Representatives, later applied to the Electoral College, counts the population of each state as the whole number of white and free citizens, including indentured servants, i.e., slaves. But African-American men gained the (official, though not practical) right to vote in Amendment 15 in 1870, as part of a Republican struggle to equalize power between Northern and Southern states (a plan with a very contemporary ring). As the patriarchal system eventually came into question, women won the vote in Amendment 19 in 1920. Nevertheless, and despite changes in demographics over time, Americans still do not have universal, equal suffrage: the Electoral College system continues to favor states with small populations, predominantly rural—usually "red"—states, in the current metaphor (Collin, 2016).

The Founders understood their political world perfectly, if cynically. But, so little clairvoyant about the future of slavery and the emancipation of women, how could they have known what the country would need in an age of electronic communication, climate change, and civil rights? In fact they did *not* proclaim that what they determined to be right for the country in 1789 would be right forever. In Article 5 they specifically declared that the Constitution could be changed under specified conditions and procedures. And it has been: with the Bill of Rights, Amendments 1–10 in 1791, and 17 more times.

A system as antiquated as the Electoral College—the "presidential electors" of Article 2 of the Executive Branch—could easily be changed to provide the broadest possible democratic representation.[2] But, since no group willingly surrenders power, revisiting the Electoral College has not been seriously tried. And candidate Hillary Clinton, abiding by the existing system like Al Gore 16 years before her, accepted her loss under its terms.

Charles M. Blow (2017), in his column for *The New York Times*, wrote that Comey's pre-election antics were instrumental in delivering the nation to Trump and his corrupt cohorts.

Within that structural frame, the question still remains: how did such a highly favored, high-polling candidate lose? One of the single most damaging events of her candidacy was FBI Director James Comey's decision, 11 days before the November election, to send to Congress a brief, vague letter revealing that the FBI might have new evidence to reopen the investigation into Clinton's nongovernmental e-mail server—an investigation that had exonerated her of all but carelessness three months before.

Comey wrote the letter despite the longstanding practice of Federal law enforcement to stay silent during elections, and despite the advice of his boss, Attorney General Loretta Lynch. When, nine days later, Comey was forced to retract further investigation because none of the e-mails were in fact new, it was too late for much impact. Was Comey's unprecedented behavior specifically directed toward a woman, considered untrustworthy? Was it an example of projective identification by some hostile FBI agents, for whom he spoke, who chose to stack the deck against the Democratic candidate?

On the Republican side it became apparent soon after Trump's inauguration that Comey had remained silent concerning substantial evidence of interaction between Trump associates and Russian intelligence figures as early as the summer of 2016 (Bump, 2017). It was a sign of President Trump's anxiety that he soon fired Comey, initially claiming the reason was the FBI's mishandling of the Clinton investigation. Meanwhile, the Trump team, from initial campaign manager Paul Manafort onward, wanted to represent Hillary Clinton as the embodiment of the corrupt condition of Washington—a figure who people dislike and distrust who is now a convicted felon.

From at least July through October, Democratic e-mails were being hacked by Russian operatives and released to the press and the public in great tranches through Julian Assange of Wikileaks, to the embarrassment of the Clinton team. Subsequently the FBI has discovered that Russian cyberscammers and "troll farms" also attempted to spread misinformation ("fake news") about Clinton and her team via falsified social media accounts aimed at 21 states, including Michigan, Ohio, Pennsylvania, and Florida (Bump, 2017). The full impact on the election of Russian interference may never be known; the degree of collusion with that interference by high-ranking figures in the Trump campaign—from Michael Flynn to Donald Trump, Jr., and Jared Kushner—will not be known until special counsel Robert Mueller completes his investigation. The drip, drip, drip of the e-mail release and the "fake" internet presence surely had an effect. Meanwhile, the Trump team, from initial campaign manager Paul Manafort onward, wanted to represent Hillary Clinton as someone who was fundamentally bad and not likable or trustworthy (Balz & Rucker, 2016).

Interview with a personal friend of Hillary Clinton's

In mid-December 2016, after the immediate shock and passion of the election had died down and reflection was possible, I was granted a long telephone interview with a friend of the Clintons from Westchester County who had volunteered in six states during the campaign. To protect his privacy I shall call him "Robert." I began with the blunt question on everybody's mind: what did he think really happened to cause Hillary's loss of the election? Robert said the most important thing he had observed was that blue-collar workers were really mad, and did not feel heard. He said her pledge to continue Obama's legacy did not convey what she had intended. Some of those folks didn't like Obama, so that was not what they wanted to hear. People had lost their jobs, they didn't believe the economy was improving, employment rates didn't seem accurate to them—rather, they believed people had dropped out of the market because they hadn't been able to get jobs. Robert added that, sadly, the idea that "black lives matter" was not well received, and not heard as intended by those who felt ignored. The same was true of the campaign's support for the LGBTQ community: what was heard in the Rust Belt, according to Robert, was "white lives don't matter," and "it's better to be gay." (Of course Robert's reasoning has, in the intervening months, become conventional wisdom. After the election, it was good to hear live, immediate testimony from the field.)

Still thinking about Rust Belt residents, I asked Robert if he thought former President Bill Clinton would have been a better person to campaign for Hillary with this constituency. He responded by saying that he thought it would have made a big difference. He added that Bill Clinton had said from the beginning that there should be a strategy for the Rust Belt states, but no one—particularly not John Podesta—would listen to him. My interviewee added that he himself thought Joe Biden could also have helped in that area. Robert emphasized that it was a real loss that Bill Clinton and Joe Biden were not asked to connect with blue-collar workers more.

The way Robert saw it, a "confluence of energies" led to the upset. But he shared a personal feeling about the campaign itself; it went something like this:

"A good lady was misrepresented by the members of her campaign staff. Hillary cares deeply about veterans and their families, I know she does, but plenty of veterans are mad at her, which is hard to explain." He added that,

> the people who are trying to make ends meet, the mother that you see in commercials who manages to hurriedly get her children to school only to run

to job one and then to job two, just didn't get the message that childcare for working mothers really matters to Hillary. We talked many times about this issue, and I know she cared, she was passionate about it—but it wasn't a big enough part of the conversation.

Robert also thought that, while it's good to have young people involved, the 30-year-old staffers were dismissive of what the 60-year-olds had to say about important voices. He said, "They were focused on the latest rock star who had endorsed Hillary, but the problem was that some of the people I was talking about didn't even know about these stars, and they just didn't care about concerts."

As we ended the conversation with thoughts about the future, Robert commented that center-right columnist Michael Barone (2016) had hit the nail on the head that day in an article entitled "Free Advice for Democrats." I rushed to find the Barone piece on Real Clear Politics. Its message was straightforward: anyone who wanted to get the Democrats on the right track needed to get out of Washington. He recommended Justice Louis Brandeis's advice from the 1930s, which was to get out of Washington, to flee the rarefied coastal climates, and put down roots in the "real" America—not university towns but the country's true heartland.

Barone too suggested that the campaign had focused on the wrong message. Instead of placing all of its energy on the ascendancy model (focusing on people on the rise), it should have spent more time focusing on the areas where people felt they were sinking.

Whose fault?

As the election receded in time, both political analysts and I have thought and written more deeply about the reasons—beyond working-class hostility—why Hillary Clinton's campaign won three million votes but did not fully succeed. Many factors contributed: it was dumb to call people "deplorables." Clinton herself has written, in *What Happened* (2017), about the damage done by constant media harping about her private e-mail server from her Secretary of State days, about the extensive focus on the Clinton Foundation's money raising that led to charges of corruption, and about latent misogyny among the public, including critical judgments that were not applied to Mr. Trump. Clinton's speeches often touched on the "historic" nature of her candidacy and made a strong appeal to women, a tactic that fanned the flames of misogyny. Of course Clinton—accurately—blames Trump's misleading, often sexist rhetoric, his looming behind her in the second debate, and his outrageous, bombastic claims for his ephemeral policies.

If we were to start impeachment proceedings, she told *USA Today*'s video newsmaker series, we must do so only after all the evidence had been gathered.

Donna Brazile, who led the Democratic National Committee during the most tumultuous days of the 2016 campaign, said that revelations about Russian meddling make her "absolutely" question the legitimacy of Donald Trump's election. Her comments prompted a Trump tweetstorm in which he pronounced Clinton "crooked" and the sorriest loser of all time. Her inability to stop talking to the media only benefited the Republican party, he added, advising her to get back to her own life and try again in three years.

The DNC meeting in February 2017 laid primary blame for the shocking loss of Clinton's focus in speeches on Trump's lack of qualifications rather than her own policies and proposals for the future. Instead of discussing the issues that were important to her, Hillary defended herself by attacking Trump's preparedness—thus ceding him the floor.

Hillary's first no-holds-barred attack on Donald Trump, which took place five days before the California Democratic primary, was described respectively by *The New York Times*, *CNN*, and *Politico* as "an evisceration," a "blistering attack," and an instance in which she "slammed" him.

Increasingly, her speeches attacked Trump; they were hardly wrong, but they created opposition and inflamed him. In short, choosing a campaign staff that favored the young, the female, and the enthusiastic whose experience may have been local or issue-oriented over "old pros" had costs as well as benefits for Clinton. The social media expertise of the two Obama campaigns, for instance, seemed to have dissipated in 2016 and was replaced by verbal attacks.

But Comey's on-again-off-again investigation of e-mails, Russian intervention in the communications sphere, and mistakes in campaign strategy do not comprise the entire explanation for Hillary Clinton's loss. The sheer opposition to a woman candidate goes deeper. Clinton had spent 50 years controlling herself, initially in Arkansas, in order not to be seen as shrill or strident, not to threaten fragile or insecure men, not to appear affected by snide critiques of her hairstyles and hairbands, her legs, her pantsuits. No male politician has to cope with these vulnerabilities simply to step into the public arena. The "haters" had been there at least since Bill Clinton's first presidential campaign; now they were happy to deride her as immoral, deeply corrupt, criminal, evil, even treasonous in the matter of Benghazi. It is hardly surprising that she was seen, even by admirers, to be guarded and to rely on an inner circle. Thus, in Donald Trump's rallies and in debates between the candidates, he could use relentless berating and dismissal of her character and her gender—to wild applause. The barrage of name-calling ("Crooked Hillary") and other unprofessional comments, such as those he used when referring to Hillary's bathroom attendance, unprecedented in modern American politics, must have been a direct blow to Clinton's psychological balance.

Feminism and me

I arrived in this world too late to know what it was like to be a woman who could not vote, and my life has been reasonably free of gender discrimination. Of course I can say that only because of the women who came before me who suffered, then took important stands on many fronts. They made sacrifices so I can vote, so I can have a career, so I do not have to be isolated as housekeeper and cook, and many more beneficial advances. I never felt I had to go down a certain path because I was a girl; the world was free for me to discover. Because women before me paved the way, I had a life where I did not feel like a second-class person because I was female. During my lifetime women have made great strides: most women I know can strive for any aspiration they choose. Before the current administration began its reign, women could actually achieve their goals.

As a young woman in Washington I met some of the people who had been leaders in the Women's Movement in the '60s and '70s. In the halls of academe I gained cognitive awareness of what women had endured since time immemorial. But I was not personally touched by a sense of being "less than." From an experiential perspective, throughout my professional training in psychology and psychoanalysis, I did not know what it was like to be disrespected as a woman. To my knowledge, I never failed to get a job because of my gender, and I have generally made as much as men in similar jobs in my field. In short, I felt equal to the men I encountered and with whom I worked. What happened to Hillary in 2016 was a stunning wake-up call for me as well as for most women I know (or know of)—popular news commentators, women in political positions, university women, and so forth.

Donald Trump emerges

Women were progressing, when, to the astonishment of many women (as well as that of Democrats in general), along came Donald Trump. In the presidential campaign of 2015–16, he expressed a brand of rudeness, vulgarity, and disrespect that had never been seen in public life. He appeared to say whatever popped into his head without any filter or judgment. Even though Mr. Trump had offered similar views about women in the past, people paid little attention to him until he rose to power. In *Trump: The Art of the Comeback*, published in 1997, he expressed a curious kind of praise for the strength of women, in his unmistakable voice. To paraphrase:

In his formative years, Trump had always believed that aggression, sex drive, and all that they entail belonged to the realm of the male. As he matured, he came to see that women far outstripped men with regard to strength, and to sex drive—and sheer ferocity. There are women, he says, who play the part of the weaker sex, who present themselves as helpless and coy, but this is a farce. Trump loves women, he assures us, but they are quite different than the way in which society depicts them: in addition to being "far worse" than men, they can be much more aggressive and certainly wily. Give credit where credit is due, he says, and pay homage to the "tremendous power" of women, which the majority of men are reticent to admit they possess.

References to unnamed body parts, that concessive claim to "love" women, anxiety about women's sex drive, aggression, and manipulative seduction—these are vintage Trump. But nothing could have prepared the world for his constant crude and lewd comments on the campaign trail and in his presidency that followed. This was magnified by video clips relentlessly shown on television. Below is a variety of those observations, from the personal to the political or policy-oriented, directed at Hillary Clinton, others, or all women:

- Referring to women as "fat pigs," "dogs," and "slobs" (or in Carly Fiorina's case, as "that nasty woman." His attack on her was personal: "Look at that face! Would anyone vote for that? Can you imagine that, the face of our next president?") (Zimmerman, 2015).
- Calling breastfeeding women, and in Hillary Clinton's case, the need for a bathroom break during a debate, "disgusting." (Trump is known to be a hand-washing germaphobe. Bodily fluids bother him.) (Diamond, 2015).
- Treating female reporters with disrespect, calling them "lightweights" and "bimbos." In Megyn Kelly's case, Trump referred to bleeding from "whatever part of her body"; after the election, in Mika Brezinski's case, when she'd been a guest at Mar-a-Lago, he falsely claimed that she was "bleeding badly from a face-lift"—female blood seems particularly to bother him (Lewis, 2016).
- Using unnecessarily sexual language to express a woman's election loss: "She got schlonged," Trump said of Clinton's 2008 defeat (Moyer, 2015).
- Bragging to a male reporter—in the infamous *Access Hollywood* tape, thinking he was off-mike—that personal celebrity means you can assault women sexually ("grab 'em by the pussy"), unchecked by any resistance (Clawson, 2017).
- Implying that military sexual assault is a natural byproduct of having men and women in the same place (Gray, 2016).
- Inciting his supporters to assault—verbally and even physically—a young black female protester at a Trump rally (Gray, 2016).
- Proposing to limit access to health care by repealing the Affordable Care Act, which disproportionately helps women and children. (A reminder to Trump and his administration: "American women" doesn't only mean White, right-wing American women who hold conservative ideologies.) (Gray, 2016).

And then there was the "lock her up" chant that must have been very distressing to Hillary and her team, not only because it was said, but also due to the fact that it gathered momentum and seemed to continue throughout the rest of the campaign.

One example was when Chris Christie neared the end of his speech at the Republican National Convention. In a protracted attack on Clinton he enumerated the many mistakes he believed she had made while Secretary of State. After each he would pause and ask the crowd to deliver a verdict of "guilty" or "not guilty." In each instance the crowd roared back "guilty" (Stevenson, 2016).

After rereading these examples of Trump's misogyny, I find it difficult to believe that anyone has consciously accepted this throwback to an attitude about women and their roles that permeated the landscape in America in the 1950s. Yet the digital airwaves continue to be filled with words, and probably feelings, of hatred, prejudice, bigotry, and racism. A shift occurred right before our eyes.

In his 2016 Plenary Address to the American Psychoanalytic Association, Donald Moss (2016) had some sobering things to say. He referred to the time in which we live as dark indeed, and went on to say that things we have taken for granted—historical progress, civilizations remaining cohesive, thought remaining relevant—are now imperiled. He said that both organized and singly operating predators are on the rise and depicted our time as that of desperate people, a destroyed planet, of "madmen and dragons."

The dignity of human beings in civil society has been altered in a fundamental way by Mr. Trump's election. The angry and distressed blue-collar workers, especially men, who followed his call have been duped: Trump promised them desired outcomes (like coal-mining or factory jobs) that he cannot possibly deliver—the pot of gold at the end of a rainbow. Do I think all the men in Ohio, Michigan, Pennsylvania, and elsewhere who voted for Mr. Trump are misogynist, scornful, sexual harassers? Of course not! Many of them, I imagine, are "decent, church-going" members of their communities who teach their children to be honest and respectful. Filled with a sense of loss, anguish, even humiliation, they need someone to blame. In hate-filled messages, Mr. Trump offered them "corrupt, crooked" Hillary, and with her all women as targets for laughter and jeers. It was a massive projection of his own animosity.

Donald Trump's treatment of Hillary Clinton during the presidential campaign was emotionally and psychologically abusive. At the very least, it was verbal violence. But Trump is capable of more than that. More than a dozen women have announced that he was physically abusive to them in his professional life over a 20-year period. Why has that abuse been tolerated? Some of the remarks Trump made in the campaign would never be tolerated in the workplace. You can't threaten people, and you can't shame them, without repercussions.

After *Fox News* executive Roger Ailes was fired in the early summer of 2016, then *Fox* host Bill O'Reilly in the spring of 2017, then Harvey Weinstein, then Mark Halperin, then an avalanche of others, no male boss should dare to say these things—or far worse—to a woman who works for him. In a 2017 *New York Times* article aptly titled "The Men Who Cost Clinton the Election," Jill Filipovic described the manner in which Matt Lauer and Charlie Rose questioned Clinton as cold and attacking; they spoke down to her, interrupted her, portrayed her as untrustworthy (when questioning Trump in the same debate, Lauer's approach was altogether different). These two men, in Filipovic's opinion, held a dim view of women who pursue power rather than remaining in the role of compliant sex objects.

As reported by the University of Michigan (2009), the definition of emotional abuse includes specific behavioral elements:

- The man says mean things to the woman.
- He doesn't let her make decisions and tells her that her decisions are bad.
- He blames, then threatens her for minor missteps.
- He yells and swears.
- He isolates her from friends and family.
- He ignores or ridicules her feelings.
- He "puts her down," calls her names, and insults her.
- He does things intended to make her feel crazy (he "gaslights" her, in 21st-century vernacular) and tells her and others that she's crazy ("Stop Abuse").

Clinton's defeat: a psychoanalytic perspective

In the presidential campaign, I believe Mr. Trump was projecting his unconscious insecurities, his distrust, his distaste for female bodies, even fear of women, onto Hillary Clinton—in verbal violence that constitutes emotional abuse. I describe the process of projective identification as it applies more broadly in various places in this book, but I will begin the conversation here. When employing this mental mechanism, a person unconsciously rids him- or herself of some aspect of the self that is intolerable. In the process, this quality or behavior is projected onto another person. Hence, it feels to the original projector that that which was "dispatched" is gone. The end result is that the first person has gotten rid of a personal attribute or quality that he or she does not like and is thereafter relieved to feel free of it. In the projector's mind, it has become a characteristic that the other unwitting person now exhibits. The recipient may or may not feel the volley that has been projected her or his way.

As an example, suppose that, as a child, a person was told that he or she was dirty, maybe even smelly. That would evoke feelings of shame in the child, and shame is hard to tolerate. It feels really bad. (There is also a tendency to hide the undesired quality, sometimes literally but most often internally.) In a relationship later in life, the former child could accuse a partner of having poor personal hygiene. An argument will ensue as the accused partner either identifies with what was said and feels ashamed or fights against an accusation that feels absurd. When opposition occurs, the projector is reinforced in feeling that lack of cleanliness is really about the other person and not about him- or herself; he or she has unconsciously dispelled any perceived tendency to be unclean.

Strong, high-status women, if they have support from friends and colleagues, are often able to deflect these volleys of spite. Donald Trump's vilification of women did not end with Hillary Clinton and the 2016 campaign—about which he remained obsessed for more than a year after his non-popular victory. After

Hurricane Maria hit Puerto Rico in 2017, San Juan mayor Carmen Yulín Cruz said that an insult from President Trump could be considered a mark of distinction. Having lived in the continental U.S. for 12 years, she continued, had taught her that there is a world of difference between a big-hearted nation and a big-mouthed president who ill-treats anyone whose thoughts, beliefs, or actions are not aligned with his expectations (Anderson, 2017).

On December 13, 2017, Mr. Trump railed against another new opponent, venting his rage at Senator Kirsten Gillibrand (Democrat, New York), who had called for his resignation. In a tweet, Trump essentially implied that Senator Gillibrand had used sex to secure campaign contributions. However, he underscored her lack of professional ability rather than depicting her as alluring. The gist of his message to women is that they can only secure success if they play the seductress; being intelligent, informed, and readily surmounting difficulty will not do the trick. There is a reason, says Thomas (2017), that powerful women are so often accused of having "slept their way to the top."

As previously mentioned, in an interview he gave to the London *Times* (Pavia, 2017), John Zinner, a clinical professor at George Washington University who also has a private psychiatric practice, said that President Trump's unchecked authority to deploy nuclear weapons at whim poses a threat to our very existence. The character of Donald Trump is, in his opinion, well known to people in the mental health field. At its foundation is a self-esteem problem that is accompanied by a sense of the grandiose. This is borne out by the names he called James Comey upon firing him ("grandstander," "showboat") and those he used for other opponents including "weak," "failure," "liar," and "loser." These four words he frequently employs, which are projected images of himself, of traits he is unable to tolerate within himself. Again, Mr. Trump, in using these names, is engaging in projective identification, as suggested in the article by Pavia (2017).

The language of defense against anxiety is a clear signal to a skilled practitioner. Women are, of course, not the only recipients of projective identification. We do not know how either the firing or the subsequent name-calling affected Mr. Comey personally, although his occasional tweets have been wryly dignified. He might have been devastated, believing that there was some validity to the negative things Mr. Trump said. He might have "considered the source," thinking the President was indulging his usual habit when frustrated: an unfiltered spewing of whatever comes to mind.

The habit of denigrating opponents is not new to Mr. Trump. We can only surmise where in his life's experience it came from. Readers who know his biography will remember reports of a calm, rather distant mother and a very demanding father with high expectations. Did Donald Trump learn in that household to regard others—at least men—as his equals, with thoughts and emotions to be acknowledged? What in his early life caused him to cast women as frightening enemies, especially with such violent language as he habitually uses?

Women fight back

Given the shock, pain, and despair of the November election, it was tremendously empowering to join the Women's March in Washington—which was simultaneously held at 673 other sites around the country—on Saturday, January 21, 2017, the day after President Trump's inauguration. Some 500,000 women and their allies (more than twice the anticipated number) filled the Mall and the surrounding blocks in a cheering rebuttal.

During one of the keynote speeches Gloria Steinem (2017) said that Trump had found a fox for every chicken coop in Washington, and warned against a Twitter finger becoming a trigger finger. She went on to say that a number of very seasoned doctors from the American Psychiatric Association have concluded that "his widely reported symptoms of mental instability, including grandiosity, impulsivity, hypersensitivity to slights or criticisms, and an apparent inability to distinguish between fantasy and reality, lead us to question his fitness for the immense responsibilities of the office."

In Virginia there is a record number of women in the House of Delegates: 12 from 2018, plus the 16 already in residence. (Watts, cited in D. Toscano, 2018). As of February 2019 there are 127 women in the US Congress.

Notes

1 Scholars trace the origins of the Electoral College back to the Romans prior to 300 BCE, an elite society well known to the better-educated Founders who had been steeped in Latin and classical history.
2 Politically sophisticated people explain that opening the Constitution to amendment, in the current climate, would offer opportunities to those who favor a wide variety of amendments—to require balanced budgets, for instance, or to forbid all abortions. Cautious politicians, under either party, can prevent an amendment on the Electoral College from even reaching the floor. Not only self-interest but the influence of their constituents prevents them from making truly democratic change.

   As of 2018, the most plausible scenario for working around the College to achieve greater democracy in presidential voting seems to be the National Popular Vote Interstate Compact, in which individual states pledge to award their electoral votes to the winner of the national popular vote if the total electoral votes in the compact reaches at least 270. The states must coordinate; to date, only ten states and the District of Columbia have agreed to the Compact.

References

Anderson, J. L. (2017, October 12). The major of San Juan on Trump's big mouth and what Puerto Rico needs. *New Yorker*.

Balz, D. & Rucker, P. (2016, November 9). How Donald Trump won: The insiders tell their story. *The Washington Post*.

Barone, M. (2016, December 13). Some free advice for the Democratic Party. RealClearPolitics.com.

Blow, C. (2017, May 22). Blood in the water. *The New York Times*.

Bump, P. (2017). Timeline: We know about Trump's campaign, Russia, and the investigation of the two. *The Washington Post*.

Clawson, L. (2017, November 27). Trump now denies "grab 'em by the pussy" recording was him, because that's how big a liar he is. *Daily Kos*.

Clinton, H. R. (2017). *What happened*. New York, NY: Simon & Schuster.

Collin, K. (2016, November 17). The electoral college badly distorts the vote. And it's going to get worse. *The Washington Post*.

Diamond, J. (2015, July 29). Lawyer: Donald Trump called me "disgusting" for request to pump breast milk. *CNN*.

Gray, E. (2016, March 2). 16 Reasons Donald Trump is definitely not "really good for women." *Huffington Post*.

Lewis, P. (2016, January 27). Megyn Kelly: The journalist who dinged Trump's ego—And got under his skin. *The Guardian*.

Moss, D. (2016). The insane look of the bewildered half-broken animal. *Journal of the American Psychoanalytic Association, 64*(2), 345–360.

Moyer, J. W. (2015, December 22). Donald Trump's "schlonged": A linguistic investigation. *The Washington Post*.

Pavia, W. (2017, May 20). The psychiatrists' verdict: Donald Trump is a man incapable of guilt, with inner rage. *The Times*.

Steinem. (2017, January 21). Here's the full transcript of Gloria Steinem's historic women's March speech. *ELLE*.

Stevenson, P. (2016, November 22). A brief history of the "Lock her up!" chant by Trump supporters against Clinton. *The Washington Post*.

Thomas, G. (2017, December 13). Trump's shameless slur against Kirsten Gillibrand. *The New York Times*.

Toscano, D. (2018). Women in the Virginia House of Delegates. Davidtoscano.com.

Trump, D. J. & Bohner, K. (1997). *Trump: The art of the comeback*. New York, NY: Times Books.

University of Michigan. (2009). *Stop abuse*.

Zimmerman, N. (2015, September 9). Trump mocks Fiorina's physical appearance: "Look at that face!" *The Hill*.

PART III

Groups of women who have been damaged

The effects of projective identification in groups

6

THE DIAL PAINTERS AND THEIR FATE

Illness and death for many

Young women were hired as dial painters in America from 1917 to 1927. They worked without knowing the dangers that were caused by radium. In industrial but studio-like settings—unlike factory assembly lines—where the original domestic glow-in-the-dark dials were created, the majority of workers were female. Many 21st-century readers will be surprised to hear that these jobs were frequently advertised in gender-segregated classified sections of newspapers indicating that "girls" were wanted for jobs in the dial-making industry (Clark, 1997). That being said, the dial painters thought they were lucky because they could earn more than $350 a week, which by today's standards would be a wage equivalent to $40,000 annually. In addition to the salary, these young women also thought they were helping the war effort by providing soldiers with glow-in-the-dark watches, something they thought would help them navigate more efficiently at night (Fonrouge, 2017). Perhaps the appeal of producing cutting-edge technology was also enticing. Some licked the ends of their brushes to create a more pointed tip more suited to the fine work (Clark, 1997). In a factory in Illinois, some enjoyed painting their fingernails with the light-green paint. After a few weeks or months at work, the girls at any radium-dial workplace became literally luminous—to the delight of some.

After I began exploring the life consequences for these women who participated in the production of radium-infused dials, I learned about the upcoming publication of Kate Moore's book, *Radium Girls* (2017), the first research study to be focused not on science, law, or commerce but on the lives and losses of individual women, which she found out about through letters and diaries in archives or family closets and by interviewing family members. Everything I learned about these women encouraged me to continue my investigation of the lives she chronicled.

This story could be told through the lens of scientific innovation or through the lens of unfettered capitalist greed, but I will tell it in honor of the trusting nature, unbearable pain, and eventual legacy in occupational law of dozens of dying women who cared deeply about having laws changed so that future generations of women would not have to suffer the same atrocities they had suffered (Moore, 2017). Moore retrieved stories of 17 women in Orange, New Jersey, and 13 in Ottawa, Illinois. They were from working-class or lower-middle-class families. When they first went to work they were very young, often right out of high school or even grammar school, the majority between the ages of 15 to 21, but occasionally as young as 12 or as old as 45. They were the children of immigrants (Albina Larice, Amelia Maggia, Edna Bolz) or Midwesterners (Marie Becker, Peg Looney, Pearl Payne). U.S. Radium initially hired about 70 of these unsuspecting young women; Radium Dial expanded its workforce to more than 1,000 (Moore, 2017). Their demographics beg for an armchair experiment: what would Eleanor Marx have done with and for them?

The amount of radium used in dial instruments is minuscule, but that does not make it harmless. In the early days in Orange, New Jersey, no managers offered even the blandest warning about safety to the women who worked there. In fact, they were told that ingestion was no problem and might even be beneficial to their appearance and health. For the best, clean-edged results, they were specifically trained to moisten and shape into a fine point, using lips and tongue, the camel-hair brushes with which they worked. The process, referred to as "lip-pointing," was passed down from one employee to the next (Moore, 2017).

Radium poisoning is not quickly apparent; symptoms take substantial time to manifest. But the women gradually developed unusual but similar conditions that could not be medically explained. First their teeth became abscessed, leaked pus, and started falling out, then chunks of their jawbones came loose in their hands (eventually labelled "necrosis of the jaw"). Some grew bulging tumors on their cheeks and chins. Some contracted cancers, most commonly sarcomas of the tibia, femur or pelvis, which caused severe limps and shrinking up to four inches. At least one bled vaginally for up to 90 days; others suffered multiple stillbirths and/or miscarriages. Excruciating back pain was practically universal. Charlotte Nevins Purcell, who chose the drastic step of the amputation of one arm in order to be able to watch her children grow up, was the rare woman to survive for many years without further damage. Instead of being able to live normal lives, have families, and grow old, most suffered a great deal and eventually died horrendous, painful deaths.

In 1924 Katherine Schaub learned from her dentist that her tooth problems might be caused by her employment; an orthodontist in Manhattan subsequently confirmed her diagnosis and that of several others. The arduous process of seeking acknowledgment and help—not, initially, money—soon began. When urged by dentists to review the issue, U.S. Radium stonewalled, beginning a long history of denial, obfuscation, and ruse. First the company employed as a paid consultant the well-known Harvard physiology professor Cecil Drinker, specialist in the inhalation of dangerous substances—along with his equally qualified wife, Dr. Katherine Drinker—to study the working conditions. The Drinkers did submit a full report to the company in June of 1924 but many of the findings were not made public and instead were withheld.

When U.S. Radium sent a copy of the report to the Department of Labor it completely omitted the health data (which the company technically owned), replacing it with statements indicating that every girl was in perfect health. As for the company president, Arthur Roeder, he ignored the recommendations the Drinkers had offered. Although Professor Drinker was angered by the use (and forgery) of his work, he ultimately agreed not to publish it. The Labor Department shelved the case. Somewhat reassured by authoritative expertise, many young women appeared to keep "drinking the Kool-Aid," by continuing to go to work at U.S. Radium. And many continued to develop horrifying unexplained symptoms (Moore, 2017).

The radium companies continued to place the same demands on the dial workers without warning them of the dangers of radium. After the Drinker fiasco in 1925, this same company, followed by other companies, hired Dr. Franklin Flinn, who examined many of the factory workers. He took blood and examined X-rays, then repeatedly told the women that they were in fine health, or that their medical issues were not caused by radiation. He even misused the instruments that detected radioactivity so they would show negative results (Moore, 2017). Later, the girls' lawyer discovered that Flinn had no license to practice medicine but instead had a doctorate in philosophy/physiology.

When radium companies did finally begin annual testing, they refused to let the women see their records for years (Moore, 2017). The women were the last to know. After Mollie Maggia became the first woman to succumb to the effects of radium in New Jersey in 1922, her family was mortified when they were told she had died of syphilis, a prognosis that, of course, they kept secret. Peg Looney of Ottawa died in 1929 of what the company doctor indicated on her death certificate was diphtheria. In spite of the mounting evidence about the lethal effects of radium, company management continued to claim it was safe. Officials knew the research indicated that radium was very dangerous—they attended a radium conference where the Eben Byers story was told (a story about a wealthy industrialist who died of radium poisoning) (Moore, 2017). Nevertheless, again and again the company lied about the dangers of radium (Moore, 2017).

The women fight back

In May 1927 the intrepid Grace Fryer, who had shrewdly left U.S. Radium to become a bank teller, helped the other women with their claims against the company. Her efforts also helped future generations of women. It had taken two years to find a lawyer brash enough to take on their case, who did not insist on upfront retainers, and who was equipped with a theory to counter their first obstacle: the short statute of limitations on "industrial accidents" in New Jersey, extended from five months to two years. That lawyer was Raymond H. Berry, and his tactics succeeded. Soon the press joined the team with headlines that graphically depicted the sickly and physically limited state of the women who were in court (Moore, 2017).

It is important to note that the radium girls eventually had help; some professionals came forward. Some dentists and doctors testified on their behalf, particularly Harrison Martland, an Orange County medical examiner who invented the two tests that definitively detected radium poisoning (Moore, 2017). Just as valuable at an early stage were civilly active, networked women with a strong social conscience, intellectual descendants of Jane Addams: Katherine Wiley, a founder of the national nonprofit Consumers League, who was alerted by a woman in the business-oriented New Jersey Department of Labor; Dr. Alice Hamilton, professionally trained in industrial toxicology; and a third woman, known to both and a skilled medical statistician, Frances Perkins. Roosevelt's secretary of labor, Perkins initiated three federal investigations (Moore, 2017). In fact, Arthur Roeder of U.S. Radium blamed "women's clubs" for all the noise (Moore, 2017). His company, of course, denied any wrongdoing and defended itself in spite of the deaths.

There also were a number of postponements and other legal irregularities that delayed proceedings in the cases against radium companies. At one point when another delay appeared to be forthcoming, one of the women's groups that was working on making sure the court case got through the system enlisted the help of Dr. Hamilton to make sure another postponement did not occur. It was at that point that well-known journalist Walter Lippmann wrote a powerful column in *The New York World* (Moore, 2017). Lippmann chastised the judicial system for delaying the proceeding of dying women who only had a small amount of money to gain at the end of their lives. Perhaps he influenced public opinion, which may have led to an eventual out-of-court settlement, providing each victim with $15,000 (equivalent to more than $200,000 today) to cover past and ongoing medical costs, and a $600-per-month annuity for life. The women who filed suits against U.S. Radium accepted the offer because most had huge medical bills and several were near death. The annuities were a good gamble for the company.

When the issues were better known in 1939, a suit in Chicago was filed on behalf of the Ottawa dial painters, argued by another bold but little-known lawyer, Leonard Grossman. Radium Dial fought it on appeals all the way to the Supreme Court, which refused to hear the case. The plaintiff did not settle; the team won a total of eight times. Catherine Donohue won the maximum award the judge could deliver.

Although these cases were thought to be victories, U.S. Radium and Radium Dial subsequently moved, changed names, hid assets, and/or went bankrupt. Hence, only the earliest plaintiffs ever collected much on their judgments.

Victimized while female

Some people said the deaths were accidental, but that was not true. As early as 1912, officials who managed radium factories knew of the dangers of radium (Hersher, 2014). In radium factories in New Jersey and Illinois, the "lip-pointing" method was used because it helped workers more efficiently gather the product. This technique also allowed them to work more quickly. There were better choices in terms of technique that could have been employed, such as those used in Europe, where "lip-pointing" was not used, but since safer practices no doubt added costs, in America these other options were ignored. From the very beginning of U.S. Radium's operations, the (male, educated upper-middle-class) chemists and engineers who worked in the laboratories—scientists, with some grasp of the dangers of exposure—were issued protective masks, gloves, and ivory forceps to use when handling tubes of radium (Moore, 2017). Where possible they stood behind lead screens, and in other settings wore lead-lined aprons. For its medical and professional staff, U.S. Radium even printed articles detailing injurious effects. In short, educated men in managerial positions mattered in the world; working-class women, easily replaceable, were no loss to society. When Kate Moore was asked, in an interview with Sarah Zhang in *The Atlantic* magazine (March 2017), whether she thought the company's management knew about the highly toxic nature of radium, she said that she did believe they thought the radium workers were expendable (Moore, quoted in Zhang, 2017).

No amount of money could recompense the women workers for their pain and suffering, or for the indifference and loss of dignity they suffered at the hands of employers they trusted. The way the corporate officials handled the situation with the female radium workers is another example of projective identification. If they had feelings and thoughts about what they were doing to the radium workers, they projected them onto the women, therefore ridding themselves of guilt and responsibility. In order to keep their fantasies alive, they monitored these young women to make sure they continued to produce more and more watches regardless of the risks. Some of them also disparaged the women who worked in the factories. For example, when the president of the Radium Corporation, Arthur Roeder, was asked in court the name of the first case he knew about, he said he didn't remember. This appears to be a very disrespectful response. The woman gave her life because of the company's failure to warn her about the lethal effects of radium and the president, who presumably prepared for the trial, couldn't even remember her name (Zhang, 2017). In another instance, the doctor (the one who did not have a medical degree) remarked that one of the women had no class because she didn't physically go to his office for an appointment when she was probably too ill to walk and was actually dying (Moore, 2017).

At one point, the Radium Dial Corporation didn't appear to care what the public or the press thought about what happened to the women at its company.

The Chicago Daily reported in its headlines a statement that illustrated the company's lack of empathy. By 1935 the company did not even deny responsibility for the deaths of the women who succumbed and instead said essentially if it were true, it was no big deal (Moore, 2017). Hence, the mechanisms they employed to disavow their part in the treatment of the women in the radium factories must have kept the guilt for their horrendous deaths at bay.

They died awful deaths

When first introduced on the market, radium was advertised as a wondrous product with a multitude of uses. It was, however, prohibitively expensive, well out of reach of the average young woman. Its price in the early 1920s was $120,000 per gram; calibrated to today's equivalent that would be around $2.2 million. Early reports of girls working in radium factories might have made it sound that they handled the element without concern, but many, realizing that in other countries the "lip-pointing" technique was not employed, inquired into its safety. Company officials repeatedly spoke of the benefits of this wonder product. Before long, the atmosphere at these factories was saturated with radium particles.

Production went on unchecked even when many of these women and girls began to display peculiar and enfeebling health problems: so ravaged was Molly Maggia's jawbone that a dentist was able to remove it using only his fingers; Peg Looney also suffered a slow, excruciating decline until she died, to the horror and grief of her family. Reports have it that Looney extracted some of her teeth herself in addition to a portion of her jawbone. A pair of tumors the size of footballs were found in Irene La Porte, who perished in 1931; a doctor claimed he was able to perform surgery on her without cutting her open. The appalling illness and deaths went on.

Public outcomes

The landmark cases of the "radium girls" set a precedent. For the first time, workers were able to receive compensation for injuries that occurred on the job. The first industrial health-reform bill was also passed by Congress in 1949 (Clark, 1997).

At the height of the Cold War, in light of ongoing nuclear research, the Atomic Energy Commission decided that the experience of the radium girls could teach science much about the effects of radioactivity over time. The commission established the Center for Human Radiobiology; research began in New Jersey and Illinois, but soon the Center merged with the Argonne National Laboratory near Chicago. The medical files of the radium girls were said to have been very valuable for research purposes (Moore, 2017). Scientists contacted as many of the living former dial painters as wished to participate, and for the rest of their lives conducted the most advanced measurements, studies, and data collection. The project operated from 1968 until 1993, and at its end had full information, including tissue samples, on 2,403 cases.

The old, old story

Kate Moore (2017) concluded her book by giving a sense of what the workers experienced in spite of all of the illness and growing awareness of the dangers of radium. One indicated that radium was used freely as though they were decorating some type of dessert with no further guidance from the company (Moore, 2017). When some employees claimed they had not been informed of the dangers of radium, the company's management indicated they had discontinued the use of lip-pointing, which was supposed to eliminate the problem. Of course that was not the case; the workers died horrible deaths.

While the Radium Dial Company finally officially went out of business through some murky dealings in 1934, another company, Luminous Processes, promptly took over business four blocks away in Ottawa and, under the same president, John A. Kelly, continued to make fluorescent-dial watches with radium. For years, radium use went uncontrolled in other, smaller sites around the United States and Canada (some near Boston, specifically Watertown and Waltham, have particular relevance for me, which will be explained later in this chapter). In the 1930s and '40s there was of course no nightly news on television, nor did national newspapers exist. Women workers in small operations far from New York or Chicago probably never saw information about their female colleagues who had suffered excruciating deaths. They almost certainly did not have the resources—or the daring and persistence—to go to court. Perhaps they had employers with integrity, who preserved their safety or compensated them for loss (Moore, 2017).

The commercial use of radium did not cease completely until the 1960s. I can only hope that the costly experience with the radium girls—together, of course, with regulation by the Federal Occupational Safety and Health Administration (OSHA), established in 1970—brought the postwar companies to introduce very scrupulous safety processes. If their employees did suffer the illness, pain, and death of the women in New Jersey and Illinois, they may never have known what was happening. Crimes against workers, especially women, are often covered up. So it was with radium: the initial multiple denials, the long court battle, finally "winning" in court; and then silent erasure. Ottawa, IL, remained a significant Superfund cleanup site in 2009, a sign both of a worthwhile national commitment to dealing with toxic waste and of the length of time such dangers can linger (Moore, 2017).

A mysterious death in the family

The pain, and the secrecy, surrounding death from an environmentally caused cancer has a complex resonance for me. When I was about seven, I discovered my beloved mother crying one day. Soon I learned that my mother's baby sister, Anna, whom she loved deeply, had been diagnosed with leukemia. Then I found out we were going to Connecticut. It was only my second trip "up North," an adventure for me although I was intermittently sad for my mother. Upon arrival on my mother's family stomping grounds, I greatly enjoyed my cousins, who showed me the ropes, exposing me to New England fun, so different from my Florida Keys explorations. There were lovely lady slippers in the woods, the joy of catching lightning bugs that I learned could be put in jars, and the scary process of getting chickens from farm to table.

As weeks turned into a month, however, I realized the situation was bad; leukemia meant that my aunt was really very sick. My mother told me that my aunt was going to die. I wasn't that sad for myself (I'd never met my aunt), but very sad for my mother, who was losing her baby sister. I listened intently to the conversations about Anna's illness and the air of suspense that surrounded it. The adults thought that Anna's cancer might be connected to the "factory" where she had worked during and after the war. They said it was radiation sickness. I don't know if my Aunt Anna worked in a radium factory or if she had been a "radium girl." I do know that I never forgot that summer when my mother was so bereft and my relatives talked about radiation, including the possibility that it was in the very popular commercial Fiestaware dishes they used. (Later it turned out that those relatives' early version of Fiestaware did indeed contain radioactive components.) It was confusing and mysterious to me.

I was intermittently sad when I saw my mother cry, but mostly I felt very lucky that summer. My cousin Patti, unimaginably, would not have a mother to go to her high school graduation, Ken would have no one to help with his homework, and Katie was too sad to talk. My uncle Jack, whom everyone said treated Anna as if she were a princess, had his sweetheart taken away. But I got on the train, headed back to my haunts in the Keys with my mother's arm around me and my father eagerly waiting at the train station. I had escaped the frightening dangers of the North; my world was intact, and I felt safe.

References

Clark, C. (1997). *Radium girls, women and industrial health reform: 1910–1935*. Chapel Hill, NC: University of North Carolina Press.

Fonrouge, G. (2017, March 22). Skin glowing from radium, ghost girls died for a greater cause. *New York Post*.

Hersher, R. (2014, December 28). Mae Keane, one of the last "radium girls," dies at 107. *National Public Radio, Incorporated*.

Moore, K. (2017). *Radium girls: The dark story of America's shining women*. Naperville, IL: Sourcebooks.

Zhang, S., interview with Moore, K. (2017, March 1). The girls with radioactive bones. *The Atlantic*, n.p.

7
THE WASP OF WORLD WAR II
Does the stigma linger?

Prior to the formation of women units in the armed services, female pilots were part of early aviation. By 1929, 75 women had acquired their pilot's licenses. Racers and performers of stunts such as Amelia Earhart and Jacqueline "Jackie" Cochran were public figures and record setters in the world of early aviation, appearing in such publications as *Life* and *Look*. On August 18, 1929, 22 competitors in a women's air derby set out from Santa Monica to Cleveland, navigating by road maps and railroad tracks alone. Fourteen completed the derby, with Louise Thaden as the winner (*Breaking Through the Clouds*, 2018).

In 1937, Jackie Cochran was the only female participant in the Bendix Air Race from Los Angeles to Cleveland, which she won by more than an hour after a risky climb above a storm in an unpressurized cockpit. Alongside her glamour, Cochran brought skill, daring, and determination to her project.

Then came Pearl Harbor. General Henry H. "Hap" Arnold, who commanded the Army Air Forces throughout the war, recognized that he desperately needed fliers for his burgeoning fleet of aircraft. Although he had to be persuaded that women pilots could help lessen the burden created by World War II, he was eventually convinced to sanction training for female aviators (Games, 2011).

Once he was finally convinced to move forward with the idea, General Arnold gave Jacqueline Cochran the job of putting together a group of women pilots. Cochran was second in fame only to Amelia Earhart in the 1930s. Her specific task was to form the Women's Air Service Pilots (WASP) unit as an experiment in September 1942 to ease the burden of male pilots.

Once established as a group of women pilots, The WASP's initial mission was to ferry the warplanes in ever-increasing production from the sites of their manufacture to the bases where they would be used or sent on to various fronts. Over two years, more than 25,000 women answered Cochran's initial call; 1,830 passed the many tests and had the flying hours required to begin Cochran's training curriculum, and 1,074 won their wings. They were chosen from candidates who had flown at least 200 hours and preferably had commercial licenses; later the required number of solo flying hours was reduced to 50. Not only was selection demanding, but the decision to enroll was far from easy. In an interview archived with the Library of Congress, Elaine Harmon recalled that she needed permission from her skeptical father to begin training as a pilot while a student at the University of Maryland (*The Guardian*, 2016).

Generally speaking, conditions confronted by this group were challenging. The flight uniforms were designed for men and therefore they did not fit them. Referred to as "zoot suits," they were far too big for smaller women, who were said to "swim" in them. Since they didn't have their own regular uniforms when not flying until April 1943, they wore white shirts and tan pants, while male officers had gabardine dress pants (Haydu, 2010).

Once in the air, conditions were not easy either, as indicated by the fact that 38 died in non-combat flight. The first woman to die was Cornelia Fort, when the wing of her BT-13 was touched by a male pilot's wing. In another case, sugar in the gas tank was the suspected cause of another death, though this was kept quiet because Jackie Cochran thought a scandal could be a threat to the corps (Nathan, 2001).

In another unfortunate incident, it was an equipment malfunction that cost the life of pilot Mabel Rawlinson, stationed at Camp Davis in North Carolina. The crash occurred when Rawlinson was returning from a nighttime training exercise with her male instructor. An eyewitness account was written by Marion Hanrahan, also a WASP at Camp Davis (Stamberg, 2010).

Rawlinson, it was believed, was trapped in the plane by a hatch that failed to deploy, while her copilot was gravely injured when he was hurled from the plane. Rawlinson was a civilian, so the military was not obliged to pay for the expenses of her death: the funeral, the sending home of her remains. Other WASP chipped in to pay for these services (Stamberg, 2010).

Since the task was so difficult, why did young women want to do it? It was a dangerous undertaking, but there were attractive aspects to such an endeavor as well. Joining the WASP gave them a chance to gain a certain type of independence that was not easy to obtain. They also met other women and formed a bond with them. Another reason seemed to be patriotism. Many women wanted to help the war effort (Games, 2011).

The women were dedicated, yet in many cases they were not treated fairly. In terms of training requirements, for example, if a woman failed a check ride, she was sent home, whereas a man who failed was dispatched to another type of training facility. There were also restrictions on talking to male pilots. Women were not allowed to talk to male pilots on check rides, but those restrictions did not apply to male pilots (Games, 2011).

They were forgotten, this group of more than 1,000 brave woman, who have been said to have been the real heroines of World War II (Haydu, 2010), ferrying planes at night in hard-to-land spaces when there were no men available to carry out dangerous missions at home (Haydu, 2010).

Success ... and consequences

The WASP were dedicated, well-trained women who went on many dangerous missions for their country. And they were successful. They completed training at a rate that matched that of men; their delivery rate was frequently better than that of their male counterparts; their rate of delivery of planes was higher than the men's rate, as was their safety rate (Nathan, 2001).

Their competence was rewarded. They were asked to train on more sophisticated and complex planes, including fighter jets such as the P-51 Mustang, the P-47 Thunderbolt, the B-17 Flying Fortress and the B-29 Superfortress bomber (the plane that was used to end the war in Japan). Two women pilots from this group took up male trainees in the B29 until a superior ended the training because he thought it was putting men to shame (Nathan, 2001).

In General Hap Arnold's farewell address he noted that the generals who commanded WASP continually called his attention to the excellent performance of these female pilots. Arnold praised the alacrity of these women who wholeheartedly carried out monotonous and routine jobs not wanted by the "hot-shot" young male pilots headed into combat or returning from an overseas tour (Haydu, 2010).

The WASP program grew beyond anyone's wildest expectation. Then, suddenly, the group was disbanded in December of 1944. Their hopes and dreams were dashed, their effort didn't matter to the powers that be. Politics trumped competence. During its two-year existence, Air Forces pilot training produced 1,074 female graduates; 916 of these women actively served in the Army Air Forces (190,000 male pilots served during World War II).The majority of the WASP were trained at Avenger Field in Sweetwater, Texas, which to this day is the sole military flying school with the status of having been intended specifically for women pilots.

During their short tenure, the WASP flew 60 million miles' worth of training and missions; delivered 12,652 planes on domestic ferrying missions and carried out various missions at nine air force bases. Because these pilots had a civilian designation, they were granted neither insurance nor military or veterans' benefits. In total, 38 WASP perished in service, 11 of those during training. But families of those fallen pilots were not permitted to place military service stars in their windows, nor were WASP given military burials—no flag for the coffin, no reimbursement for burial expenses (Merryman, 2001).

To add insult to injury, records of the services of WASP were classified, and as such were unavailable to researchers for 35 years. Not until 1973 did the Air

Force announce that it was accepting women for training as military pilots (Ghosh, 2015).

Yet, even when the "experiment" had proved so successful, the WASP were never (as General Arnold originally intended) sworn in to the military. They did not hold officer ranks or get promoted; they paid their way to their training sites, paid for their own insurance, apparently had room-and-board en route deducted from their pay (Haydu, 2003).

To add insult to injury, even though the experiment was successful, the overall outcome was a failure: women made major contributions to the war efforts in World War II but they were not treated with respect. Instead, they were summarily dismissed. Men who were pilots did not want them to be in the military, and as a result they were never sworn in. Promises made were not kept.

Part of the dismissal process: the negative media campaign

Among the most damaging things that happened to the WASP was a negative media campaign launched against them by male combat pilots (Merryman, 2001). The male civilian pilots, after uniting politically (their status as AAF cadets and trainers had allowed them to avoid the draft and given them the resources to form the lobby), asserted that the WASP had received preferential treatment; this was a ploy to deflect attention from the fact that these men refused to serve as combat soldiers, avoiding the draft because of their status as AAF cadets and trainers. The lobby launched an anti-WASP campaign in the media and Congress, a campaign that flourished due to commonly held ideas about male superiority (a year previously, similarly, the Women's Army Corps had been subject to a slander campaign). What's more, the War Department had a PR plan in place regarding the WASP—the policy of which was to sidestep media publicity because it was thought (especially if WASP deaths were to become public) that the public would be against the program. With this policy in place, the male civilian pilots' voices went uncontested (Merryman, 2001).

As stated above, the male civilian pilots' powerful lobby had the attention of the media as well as Congress, to which the pilots instigated a letter-writing campaign; behind the campaign were prominent male-run aviation associations and veterans' groups. When the pilot lobby discovered that the House Committee on Military Affairs was promoting passage of a bill to give female Air Force pilots military status, they mounted an attack against the WASP and sought to introduce a bill of their own in favor of finding positions for male pilots and keeping them from being assigned to the Army's ground forces (Merryman, 2001).

The men in Congress and the military—including all those who had opposed women aviators from the outset—won. In October 1944, each WASP received a letter thanking her for her *volunteer* help, but proclaiming that it was no longer needed as of December 20, 1944. General Arnold bureaucratically conceded that those who were still in training could finish. Thus the "Lost Last Class," as it was dubbed, graduated, but, as Landdeck (2016) tells us, served only two-and-a-half weeks before being sent home on December 20, along with all the rest of the WASP (Stamberg, 2010).

Last resting places

In 2002 the WASP returned to contemporary attention: they were dying. It took them 30 years to obtain veteran status (in 1977); most probably believed that status included the right to interment at Arlington National Cemetery. Strong investigative journalism by *The Washington Times* revealed that, in 2002, a ruling had stated that the "right" had never provided for burial of their bodies, but only for their ashes to be inurned in the Arlington columbarium. But in 2015, then-Secretary of the Army John McHugh, in an unpublicized memo, suddenly reversed course and rescinded even that privilege: no WASP burials in Arlington whatsoever. This new form of second-class treatment made things go from bad to worse.

The impact of the decision on the WASP emerged when one of their last effective spokeswomen, Elaine Harmon (who as a native Washingtonian had been active in the campaign for veteran status) died in April 2015 at age 95; her inurnment was denied. Obtaining General McHugh's ruling only under the Freedom of Information Act, her daughter, Terry Harmon, was dismayed to learn that the Army was again excluding the WASP from Arlington.

A year and a half after Harmon's death, the Army finally gave formal recognition to the equality of female pilots, and she, a former WASP, was interred alongside her fellow (male) veterans with full military honors.

I find myself wondering what today's world might be like if all women had been able to pursue the early interest in the STEM fields that motivated the young WASP to join the wartime service. Consider the African-American mathematician "computers" at NASA in Margot Lee Shatterly's book and film, pointedly titled *Hidden Figures* (2016), or earlier still, the women mathematicians who served before World War II in David Alan Grier's *When Computers Were Human* (2005). Both groups were recovered for history only in the 21st century. Had more women been recruited for science, math, and engineering, we might have had female astronaut pilots long before Eileen Collins (1991) and Sally Ride (1978).

How much have things changed?

Yes, women are now airline pilots and they are officers. They even have their own uniforms. However, one wonders how their presence is compared to the presence of men who are employed by major airlines. Are they really as valued as men who fly commercial jets? As much as one might think the plight of the WASP is no longer part of our culture, one is reminded of the dismissive treatment a talented female pilot received in April 2018.

During what was thought to be a routine fight, Tammie Jo Shults made an emergency landing at the Philadelphia International Airport and saved 149 passengers in the process. Passengers called her a hero after the plane's engine apparently blew up (Stanglin, 2018).

CNN reported the story, but said nothing of the heroine, the female pilot. In spite of Captain Shults's ability, experience, and act of heroism, the airline said that it was "devastated" about the situation yet the spokesman did not mention Shults by name (Betz, 2018).

Compare this to "Sully" Sullenberger, the pilot who landed the plane he was flying on the Hudson. Sullenberger became an instant celebrity, was appointed a role of CBS News aviation and safety expert, and became a bestselling author. Sullenberger's time is now spent as a speaker with the Harry Walker Agency and is on an advisory committee for the Department of Transportation.

This was not the first time Shults was held to a different standard. After being turned down by the air force, she served as a Navy pilot but was not able to fly combat missions since she left active duty two days before the Clinton administration was asked to allow women to be given these assignments, which were available to men for many years (Haag, 2018).

References

Associated Press. (2016, January 1). Families of female pilots from Second World War struggle for equal burial rights. *The Guardian*. Retrieved from www.theguardian.com/us-news/2016/jan/01/second-world-war-us-female-pilots-wasps-arlington-nationa-cemetery.

Betz, B. (2018, April 18). Former ace Navy pilot ID'd as hero who landed damaged Southwest flight. *Fox News*.

Breaking through the clouds: The first Women's National Air Derby (2018). Archetypal Images, LLC.

Games, B. (2011). *WASPS of WWII*. Martinville, IN: Fideli Publishing.

Ghosh, S. (2015, November 8). We salute the service of World War II WASPs. *My Central Jersey/US Today*.

Grier, D. A. (2005). *When computers were human*. Princeton, NJ: Princeton University Press.

Haag, M. (2018, April 18). Southwest pilot of Flight 1380 is Navy veteran hailed for her "nerves of steel." *The New York Times*.

Haydu, B. F. (2003). *Letters home 1944–1945: Women Airforce Service Pilots*. Riviera Beach, FL: TopLine Printing and Graphics.

Haydu, B. F. (2010). *Letters home 1944–1945: Women Airforce Service Pilots* (4th ed.). Publisher Unknown.

Landdeck, K. S. (2016, September). A woman pilot receives the military funeral the Army denied her. *The Atlantic*.

Merryman, M. (2001). *Clipped wings: The rise and fall of the Women Airforce Service Pilots (WASPs) of World War II*. New York, NY and London: New York University Press.

Nathan, A. (2001). *Yankee doodle gals: Women pilots of World War II*. Washington, DC: National Geographic Society.
Shatterly, M. L. (2016). *Hidden figures*. New York, NY: HarperCollins.
Stamberg, S. (2010, March 9). Interview with WASP Marion Hanrahan. NPR.org.
Stanglin, D. (2018, April 18). Southwest emergency landing pilot Tammie Jo Shults is a pioneer with "nerves of steel." *USA Today*.

8
THE CHALLENGE
Healing groups and cultures

In this chapter I turn my focus to the difficult question of repairing the dreadful damage that occurs when groups of people, often ethnic or cultural rivals, violently oppose one another. While it is possible to help an individual, whether the helper be a parent, friend, or therapist, a reader might justifiably wonder how change could even be attempted in the case of violence perpetrated by large groups of people, even terrorist groups. Having suggested that change is possible while in Klein's depressive position, I now explore the problems that emerge when whole cultural groups behave in an aggressively paranoid fashion. To begin with, using Klein is tricky. What she said is most often not to be taken literally but must be interpreted. To take Klein at face value can be problematic (Rasmussen & Salhani, 2010) since she was not referring to a linear construct of development but to constellations of psychological phenomena that are part of the landscape of the mind throughout life. Hence, progression in not consistently forward-moving but goes in one direction and then returns to an earlier position. Klein's theory is also complicated because while she did talk about movement from the paranoid-schizoid position to the depressive position as a developmental achievement early in life, this pattern does not remain fixed. Klein thought that during various times in life, people move back and forth between the depressive position and the paranoid-schizoid position. The idea of fluctuating mental states is important in this discussion and presents a unique perspective since it involves shifting qualities of racism and ethnic hatreds (Rasmussen & Salhani, 2010).

Proceeding cautiously without attempting to expound on all parts of Klein's theory is essential since all of her terms do not lend themselves easily to the analysis of groups. Hence, it is advisable to choose and develop concepts that can be applied to various categories of people, e.g., projective identification, a term that applies to single individuals as well as to groups. It may also be possible to combine Klein's ideas with others who are familiar with the effects of culture on groups of people.

With the aforementioned ideas in mind, one wonders how we can best understand how heads of state, ethnic, or social groups—or entire countries—can modify their behavior, to say nothing of their (or our) distorted thinking. Do some mechanisms that apply to individuals also apply to groups? Can people be brought to understand the variations of culture and ideology in our modern world, then surrender their perceived need to take hostile action—action that has untenable and long-lasting effects? Can they learn to mentalize?

After tragic conflicts occur, many well-intended people want to help. Those not trained as professionals are likely to encounter limits when attempting to significantly change a situation. The role one plays at the moment often dictates how much one can intercede. But whenever feasible, it is desirable to help others understand that all people are allowed to hold their cultural traditions, ideas, and opinions as their own, as a crucial part of compatible living. While this idea seems simple, the process is extremely difficult to achieve without a thorough understanding of the cultural traditions that have shaped the combatants.

Nevertheless, just as individuals can change, change is also possible on a large scale. Peoples with different cultural or institutional beliefs can coexist if each group makes committed efforts to respect the rights of other groups to believe what they wish without repercussions—but if, and only if, sincere attempts at mutual understanding and respect for truth are accepted as core values of each group. People can learn to understand the variations of culture and ideology in our modern world. I believe change can be created by applying the principles inherent in mentalization (see Chapter 11) to move beyond the paranoid-schizoid position of attempting to destroy despised others. If leaders in various settings can find ways to metabolize aggression on a large scale, if groups can be persuaded to "own" their aggression and mourn the loss of what cannot be, then hostile forces can collectively work toward repairing misunderstanding. They can accept the uniqueness—or at minimum, the rights—of others. Then the possibility of hope can exist. (This topic will be discussed in more detail in Chapter 12.)

An example of projective identification in groups: when mentalization failed at the Northbrook Academy

It all began during an evening graduate seminar, when an uncanny slide appeared on the screen. The class was cotaught by Dr. N (Miriam), an experienced and well-respected instructor, and her counterpart Dr. Y (Peter).

Not only had they not discussed Peter's startling slide during their seminar preparations, which was something they always did, but Miriam had never seen this incongruous slide that portrayed an altered perception of reality reminiscent of a Dali painting. She couldn't understand how it was related to the topic they were presenting that evening, and felt a bit embarrassed for Peter, whom she liked and respected as a colleague.

In an attempt to help Peter out and cover for him while he continued to fidget with the slide projector, Miriam tried to shift the focus from him and his disturbingly inappropriate slide by joking with the class about her colleague's sense of humor. The class chuckled and they moved on. Despite the odd beginning, as far as Miriam was concerned the seminar continued as usual.

Only later did she learn that, while she was getting material from her briefcase to hand out to the students, Peter (who was not a native speaker of English) had said something to one member of the group that included a racial slur. Later, when both teachers went over this incident with the class, another woman said that she, like Miriam, hadn't heard the "n-word" comment either; many, however, did.

After class ended, Miriam and Peter were chatting while waiting for the elevator when a student approached Peter. Assuming that he wanted to talk to Peter about a personal matter, Miriam started to step away, but the student said, "You can hear this too, if you want to." That invitation is how Miriam learned that, during the class, Peter had had a racially tinged verbal exchange with this very student. She was surprised and extremely concerned to learn that a student, perhaps several students, had been disturbed by the language Peter used.

When Miriam and Peter talked during the week before the next seminar, they decided they needed to address the issue right away, at the beginning of the class. No matter what Peter had intended, after all, it was clear that something negative had happened and some class members were upset. The teachers met with the students after class on two occasions, to apologize and to help them express their feelings. Further meetings were held with the curriculum chair, program chairs, and others to help the students process their experiences. In fact, the disturbing event was processed throughout the semester, and the seminar atmosphere appeared to return to normal. Although she was not guilty of saying a racist word, Miriam reported that she and Peter worked in tandem with the students to help them express themselves. She thought that by encouraging the class to discuss their feelings, she and Peter had dealt with an unfortunate situation in a thoughtful and compassionate way.

After the seminar ended that semester, however, Miriam heard at a committee meeting that some participants thought that the teachers of the class should no longer be permitted to teach at the academy because of their racist behavior. In the subsequent report, she said she was quite taken aback, adding that she thought such a drastic step was hardly reasonable, especially considering that she was innocent. The talk was all very accusatory. Her dismay was compounded by the fact that this particular committee was going on very few facts about the situation, just hallway gossip.

Miriam suspected that many academy members—despite extensive training— were distancing themselves from allegations of prejudice or bigotry by going along with an unfair and highly punitive response to the potentially "guilty" pair. Miriam thought to herself, if we don't teach our students about racism and how to avoid joining the aggression of others without knowing any facts, we are doing them a great disservice. However, instead of helping students learn the importance of thinking for themselves and rendering decisions after learning facts, the group seemed to collude with those who advocated removal of the teachers by jumping on the bandwagon, judging without actually knowing what had occurred. Projected ideas flew around the campus. In order to distance themselves from the incident, the academy's leaders raced to find a solution. Others followed the crowd by immediately judging the instructors based on hearsay. They unfortunately modeled this behavior for students. In so doing they distanced themselves from the truth.

This incident and the overwhelming response to it was clearly an example of projective identification. A portion of the faculty was projecting its aggression and possibly racism onto Peter and Miriam to rid participants of negative thoughts. These faculty members created a fantasy that the two teachers were guilty of actions that might warrant dismissal. To make a bad situation worse, consciously or unconsciously the academy's administration thought that they too had to dispel the building aggression and anger toward the teachers. Rather than tolerating the growing tension while gathering information, and only then rendering a decision, they failed to thoroughly review and assess the situation while leading with integrity and honor.

There was no hearing or even a proper interview. Peter admitted in a letter to the Board of Directors (which he shared with Miriam) that he alone had caused the problem, and that Miriam had done nothing wrong. Both teachers had taught together with positive evaluations for several years. Yet the administration formally reprimanded Dr. N (Miriam) but not Dr. Y (Peter); others in leadership positions went along with the decision or refused to get involved. Thereafter, a committee that is supposed to "right wrongs" at the academy never responded to Miriam's letter when she sought assistance. Even though Miriam was not guilty of having uttered a single racist word, she was swiftly removed from teaching. The chair of the committee that filled teaching positions for that course informed her in an email that she would not be permitted to teach at all the following year; he refused to speak with her in person or on the phone in spite of her requests. Miriam was then disenfranchised by a number of people in the larger faculty group: she became the scapegoat. At the same time, the chair of the curriculum committee told Peter that he didn't *have to* teach that seminar the next year, apparently to help distance him from the tainted incident. He was instead asked to teach two other classes.

This incident is an example of projective identification in an institute of higher learning that professes to promote the exploration of the human psyche in all its complexity for purposes of fully understanding the human experience—a position diametrically opposed to the unfair and discriminatory, hurried process that stripped Miriam of her ability to teach and deprived her of a fair-minded dialogue with peers who were not influenced by the group projective identification, the mechanism that affects those who have trouble thinking for themselves and speaking with their own voices. It is also an example of gender discrimination and harassment. The people who dealt most directly with Miriam's case were men, but women were involved as well. In this case I would say that *reverse swarming* occurred. Whereas Atwood (2017) talked about the fact that women at times will gang up on other women—"group swarming"—when referencing encounters between the "aunts" and "handmaids" in her book, it is also the case that women can desert other women. That is what appeared to happen in Miriam's case. Women who could have intervened did not. It appeared to her that they did not want to get involved either by helping her or by attacking her; instead they turned their backs on her. Rather than getting to the bottom of the incident in a thorough, fair, and just way, they put a committee together to study cultural differences.

It is not known if anything was learned from the aforementioned situation or if an opportunity for "taking back projections" aimed at Miriam occurred, but it is clear that women are subjected to such bullying and dismissal every day (men to a far lesser degree, given their long history of power). The words and behavior of President Donald J. Trump suggest that mistreatment and misogyny will continue until women truly have the same rights as men.

References

Atwood, M. (2017). Margaret Atwood on what *The Handmaid's Tale* means in the age of Trump. *The New York Times*, p. 10.

Rasmussen, B. & Salhani, D. (2010). A contemporary Kleinian contribution to understanding racism. *Social Service Review, 84*(3), 491–513.

9
THE ATROCITIES OF PHYSICAL ABUSE

Genocide and rape in Rwanda and sex-trafficked girls

The genocide and rape in Rwanda

This chapter explores how projective identification could have contributed to the 1994 genocide in Rwanda. While there are a number of factors that led to that catastrophe, projection from colonialists—first German and then, after World War II, Belgian—who had occupied their country played a major role in the conflicts between the Hutus and the Tutsis. The Rwandans thereafter projected what was originally European aggression onto each other, culminating in the slaughter of 800,000 people in 100 days (Dallaire, 2003).

There is no doubt that Europeans favored the Tutsis, in part because of their (marginally) lighter skin and greater height. Colonization in central Africa occurred near the beginning of the period of fascination with physical anthropology as a popular interest, when racial theory based on practices like caliper-measured skulls and facial features assured the "Nordic" Europeans of their superiority (Robbins, 1999). This pseudo-science justified their rule, licensed them to project their own social structures onto Africans, which resulted in the eugenics movement. In general, the Belgians thought the Tutsis were superior, which led them to insist on ID cards so they could distinguish Tutsi from Hutu. They attempted to appoint Tutsis to chieftainships, pushing other Rwandans toward a rigid caste system (Des Forges, 1999).

Moreover, socioeconomically the Tutsis, who were most often cattle owners—always a privileged status in East Africa—were thought to be richer, whereas the Hutus were cultivators or peasants and economically less secure; those distinctions were far from absolute. As the Belgians slowly departed, they left the Tutsis in a dominant position in Rwanda, making the Hutus feel like second-class citizens. Although these culturally defined identities have indeed played a big part in Rwanda's history, experts on African history say it is hard to gauge the extent of the animosity prior to the arrival of the European colonizers. Discord between the two cultures does not appear to have descended into mass murder and other atrocities until after independence. Projection from hierarchically conditioned Europeans is certainly part of the picture, as are various other projective identifications that were rooted in "badness within" that had to be expelled onto the other (or others). Hence, the phenomenon continued of having to rid oneself of unmetabolized "bizarre objects" (a term used by Bion in reference to the negative, overwhelming thoughts and feelings of a child who cannot be soothed). This discussion will be considered and broadened as it applies to the Tutsi and Hutu's slaughter of each other in the 1994 killing of 800,000 people (Dallaire, 2003).

Origins and history

How could such a thing happen in our seemingly civilized world? Did it reflect prejudice passed on from colonialists—first German and then, after World War II, Belgian—who had occupied their country? Did the Rwandans thereafter project what was originally European aggression onto each other, causing the slaughter of 800,000 people, most of them innocent? On January 11, 1994, General Dallaire wrote to Kofi Annan. He was in charge of the United Nation's peacekeeping force in New York. He reported that Jean Pierre, an anonymous informant occupying the higher inner circles of the Interahamwe Rwandan Militia, said that Hutu extremists had received an order to register all Tutsi in Kagili, and had a suspicion that this was for their extermination. He provided the example that in 20 minutes his personnel would be capable of murdering as many as 1,000 Tutsi (Dallaire, 2003).

There is no agreed-on history of early Rwanda. This is partly due to the difficulties of re-creating the history of an oral society and partly to the distorted and sometimes racist eyewitness accounts by early colonizers. But the main difficulty is the fact that the arguments over history have become important politically (Fullerton, 2011).

When the Belgians took over the rule of Rwanda after the Germans left, they viewed the minority Tutsis as closer to Europeans and elevated them to positions of power over the majority Hutu, which exacerbated the feudal state of peasant Hutus and overlord Tutsi (Dallaire, 2003).

Peter Uvin is provost and professor of political science at Amherst College and an authority on the Rwandan genocide. He has said that, in trying to understand or explain the Rwandan genocide, it is not important to know the exact history between Hutu and Tutsi. Economically, the country was ripe for revolt: in 1989 the price of coffee—the primary export commodity—had collapsed worldwide. In 1990 the IMF devalued the franc, devastating farmers. The World Bank and IMF were demanding austerity measures as the price of further aid. Tinder was waiting for a spark. But First World countries were inclined to de-emphasize their roles under the guise of old tribal tension building on the Rwandans' shared perceptions and the firm belief that the other was different—not like them—and could be set apart, regardless of the facts (Uvin, 2009). A perspective from within the Hutu-Tutsi conflict proposes that the origin of genocide is difficult to trace, elusive, emanating from cumulative grudges and misunderstandings; it was fueled by inciting slogans and by an unquestioning loyalty to those in power (Dallaire, 2003).

All too visible

The slaughter and mutilation of Rwandan Tutsis by their next-door neighbors in 1994 happened in plain sight; Hutu military leaders even broadcast instruction, as well as incitement, to the genocidaires on the radio station Milles Collines. Famously, nobody did anything about it. Unchallenged—and with UN military observers forbidden to intervene—militant Hutus enacted their fantasies in vicious ways, soldiers with guns and civilians with machetes and other daily tools. Thinking was replaced by rage at their supposed suppression, which they planned to avenge through the atrocities they committed. In the soldiers' minds, their victims were dehumanized into pure enemies. The Hutu Interahamwe convinced themselves that they were in fact superior and thus justified in killing and maiming people of lesser worth who had lorded it over them (Smyth, 1996). According to the Resource Information Center (2001), it is primarily the Interahamwe militia who were active in the 1994 Rwandan massacre. Under President Habyarimana and with the support of the Rwandan army, two militias were formed in 1992, the Interahamwe and the Impuzamugambi. They killed more than 2,000 civilians, the majority of them Tutsi.

Philip Gourevitch, who conducted a study of the genocide, said the Interahamwe militia was rooted in soccer fan clubs and a force—political, economic, and military—that became known as "Hutu Power" (Resource Information Center, 2001).

The militia also killed Hutus who defended Tutsis, and even some who simply witnessed attacks. Their crimes were soon discovered by others. The soulful general General Roméo Dallaire, commander of the UN peace force, spoke of eyewitness reports of slaughter in a church where Tutsi families had gone to hide or seek sanctuary. Priests and UN observers, he reports, came upon a grisly scene, with the bodies of hundreds of men, women, and children strewn in the aisles and pews. He tells of how the militia operated methodically, and how they laughed and joked as they went to work with their machetes. By the time the slaughter had spent itself, in 100 days, 800,000 people, Tutsis and Hutus, had been killed—truly a genocide. Perhaps three-quarters of the Tutsi population was lost.

Women in war

That number of victims, 800,000, is the iconic symbol of the Rwandan massacre, amplified by its depiction as genocide. What has been forgotten (or obscured) is the countless women who suffered rape as a weapon of war before they were killed, mutilated, or left to live in pain and shame. Rape in war is as old as organized human society, but for some two centuries it was—like most issues of perverted sexuality—suppressed in polite company and in print. The 20th century began to pull back the curtain, initially in propaganda: Belgian nuns were said to be raped at the beginning of World War I (Rizvanolli, Bean & Farnsworth, 2005).

But uneasy silence returned at the end of World War II, when women and girls in Berlin and its outskirts were raped on a massive scale by an advancing Red Army certain of its imminent victory (Johnson, 2002). Was this ugly fortnight suppressed because Russia was an ally of the West? Perhaps, but on the other side of the globe the Japanese kept brothels full of Korean "comfort women," most of whom were subject to rape, so silence prevailed in Asia for decades as well. Did many allies somehow perceive that dirty German women—wives, daughters, mothers of their dehumanized enemies—deserved this vicious punishment for what had been done to Russians and Ukrainians, among others? Projection of all the slaughter in which allied soldiers themselves had participated for more than five years is an obvious component of the Russian rampage. And hundreds of humiliated women no doubt simply chose a complicit silence, in defeat.

The first widely publicized modern use of rape as a weapon of war occurred in the Balkan Wars in the 1990s. Although atrocities were committed on all sides in this conflict of neighbors with a reputed history of religious rivalry, the media gradually told the world of Croatian and (largely) Serbian men systematically raping Bosniak women, often in prison camps, with the specific goal of impregnating them with non-Muslim children and rendering them dishonored, "untouchable" by Muslim men: genocide by other means. In the hatred, depersonalization, and violence between former neighbors, the Balkan tragedy for women is most similar to what happened in Rwanda (Neill, 2000).

Fisk tells a story of Ziba, a 26-year-old Bosniak Muslim woman who, together with about a hundred others, many with their very young children, had been confined to a school gymnasium. Inebriated Serbian militia bearing guns and grenades burst in, appraised them, and announced that since these women were clearly prolific, they were going to be made to bear more children, only these would be fathered by Chetniks (and therefore be non-Muslim). Ziba was among the first 12 to be selected from the group, the youngest of whom was just 16. Ziba was wrenched from her children, who believed she was going to be killed. The 12 were transported to a hotel in Kalinovik, where they were forced to clean the rooms and scrub the floors, after which they were given something to eat. Following the meal the militiamen ordered the women to accompany them to the hotel rooms. Ziba was taken upstairs by two men whom she describes as drunk and dirty. One of them told her that if she didn't cooperate her throat would be slit. For half an hour the two men took turns raping her. After being raped, the 12 women were brought into a common room and ordered to clean the hotel rooms again, after which they were returned to the gymnasium. Zika and the others were subjected to this ritual every day for a month: taken to the hotel, made to clean the rooms, given a meal, raped multiple times, made to clean the rooms once again, and transported back to the gymnasium.

In 2017 a similar scenario began to proliferate itself in South Sudan: soldiers of the dominant Dinka group rape the women of the Nuer if they so much as leave their refugee camps to forage for food or firewood. These rapes are in retribution for the deeds of the women's rebel husbands and sons (Ferguson, 2017).

Since the genocide, Rwandans have somehow managed to live and work together, building a successful economy and, apparently, society. Perhaps a clue as to how that happened lies in photographs taken by Pieter Hugo at the 20-year commemoration of the genocide in 2004. He went to southern Rwanda, hoping to capture images of people living together two decades afterwards, and captured a series of unlikely, almost unthinkable tableaus. In one picture a woman rests her hand on the shoulder of the man who killed her father and brothers. In another a woman poses with a casually reclining man who looted her property and whose father helped murder her husband and children. In the second photo, the perpetrator is a Hutu who was granted a pardon by the Tutsi woman who survived his crime. The images do not bring to mind happy people; there is little evidence of warmth between the pairs, yet they are there, together. A reconciliation, however uneasy, has occurred (Incredible Stories of Forgiveness, 2014).

Sex-trafficked girls/women

Child sex trafficking is rampant in the 21st century; young women are snatched from our doorsteps in every city in the United States and forced or sold into sexual exploitation. When I ask people what human trafficking means, the responses are invariably some version of one theme: "Things that they do in Africa or, no, maybe it's more like places in Asia." (Occasionally a couple of "South Americas" or "the Balkans" are tossed into the mix.) My casual survey participants usually add that bad guys kidnap young girls and put them in prostitution rings. "It's really bad; 'they' should really do something," is a frequent parting remark. As much as I might have the inclination to respond, "Are you kidding me?" I can't, because a few months ago I was saying a similar thing. But the victimization of young people is much closer than we think, a fact I learned recently when reading local accounts of trafficking.

This trauma is happening here, in front of our very eyes—where I live, in Washington, DC. Young women are being terrorized: held in fear by a kidnapper-pimp at gun- or knifepoint, often in a sleazy motel, their sexual acts surveilled, and not only their cell phones but their underwear taken away from them, a humiliating cruelty that threatens their most intimate identity. If a young woman sees the opportunity to escape, she is afraid to: she is told she'll be arrested for prostitution rather than cared for and treated. And that allegation is often true. The police, and the media, report cases only when they have successfully been uncovered by capture of a perpetrator—such as in 2016, when a Washington policeman was found to be maintaining a brothel-like apartment (Noble, 2013).

In the 21st century, sex trafficking in children is rife in the United States. Girls and young women in every city are coerced or sold into lives of sexual exploitation. Ordinary citizens have no idea of the magnitude; to reiterate, when asked to define human trafficking they tend to say it's a phenomenon that happens elsewhere—in Africa, Asia, South America, maybe the Balkans. The perception is that girls are kidnapped by "bad guys" and forced into prostitution rings. They don't realize this is happening on our very doorsteps.

What many people don't realize, if they are aware of the problem of human trafficking, is the alarming rate it has increased in the last 10 years. According to Sher (2011), it began to rise after the last recession in 2009 continuing into 2010. One example of this increase occurred with homeless young people; a rate that doubled during the same period. To make matters worse, once in the system, girls rarely go back to a wholesome family environment since they came from troubled homes in the first place (Sher, 2011). Although many young women might appear to be sophisticated due to their evening attire, they are often scared girls.

In 2016 Colbert I. King of *The Washington Post* described the situation, saying that there is little news coverage of this type of slavery; what's more, the victims suffer lifelong trauma, and often slip into addiction—which can ultimately cut their lives short. King reported that, at the end of December 2015, President Obama designated January 2016 as National Slavery and Human Trafficking Month. The President compared human trafficking to a form of modern-day slavery, proclaiming it an outrage; he said that this practice greatly undermines the cohesiveness of society and should be of concern to communities everywhere. We must, he added, work toward a future in which traffickers are made to atone for their crimes and no one is deprived of freedom and basic human dignity. Although Obama's proclamation described the mobilization of intelligence teams, law enforcement, prosecutors, technology companies and protection for the foreign-born "maids" suffering here unwillingly, such a future is on a distant horizon.

One brave young woman's story

One unusual risk-taker was 17-year-old Joanie, who lives as a prostitute near South Street Seaport. She talked to the *New York Times* crime reporter Michael Wilson in 2017. At that time, she lodged a complaint with the police and eventually testified against the man who was responsible for her captivity. Joanie's case is of particular importance as it sheds light on the problems that can befall teenagers in particular.

Disgruntled with her mother, she contacted a man (ten years older than she believed) whom she had met online and went to his Bronx apartment, where she found his partner, his two children, and two other sex slaves. After a month during which she was forced into many sexual encounters each night in return for food and shelter, she waited until he was drunk, then slipped out of the apartment and managed to find her way home (Wilson, 2017).

Joanie is among many thousands of women and children—including boys, to be sure—who, in order to survive, use their bodies to perform a wide variety of acts against their wills. If they do manage to escape, young prostitutes are often made to feel guilty for not having tried harder and earlier to free themselves from a pimp's tyranny.

Notably, Joanie did not run away to the streets, as has been true of unhappy teens for decades, and get recruited there, a victim of hunger and despair. Not only had she met the pimp online, but he advertised her, and other young women, to potential customers online—often describing them as younger still than they were. A website notorious for filling this immoral function is Backpage, characterized by the *New York Times'* Nicholas Kristof (2017) as essentially an online brothel to which nearly 75 percent of the cases of juvenile sex trafficking in the United States can be traced. Backpage has been attacked by credit card companies, by the attorney general of California, and even by a bipartisan Senate subcommittee. But few inroads have been made. Although Backpage disappeared, other "online marketplaces" will promptly materialize to fill the profitable commercial vacuum. Daniela Petrova (2016a), who reports for Salon, has learned that the children most vulnerable to sexual exploitation are those who have been abused. She describes one case who had a long history of physical and sexual abuse by her family, as well as abandonment.

The girl in question came from a loveless home, and therefore found herself susceptible to the attentions and flattery of a pimp, who showered her with gifts, said he loved her—endearments were unknown to her—and put her to work for him. Eventually she was arrested by an undercover police officer. Petrova (2016b) points out how easy it is to recruit children from unstable backgrounds (foster children, for instance) and points out that some girls initially find their way into these circumstances because they are frustrated at home and, acting out, become runaways. Once lured or coerced into prostitution, it's very difficult for these girls to extricate themselves if they're estranged from their families and have no one to call, no one to turn to for the fare of a bus ticket home.

Emotional suffering

From a mental health perspective, sex trafficking is devastating. These young women, who are often legally children, do not consider themselves victims of a crime. Instead, they feel guilty, as though they're partly to blame for what has happened to them. The exploited may begin to accept their lot in life as something they deserve. If they are angry with their families, however temporarily, that may add guilt to their negative feelings about themselves. Not only have they been violated physically, but they also suffer from mental anguish; with the intensity of youthful emotions, they think that they are flawed, that their lives are ruined, and that they participated in the process.

Human trafficking is perpetuated by shame. And where shame is, there is a wish to hide. Yet the life may look glamorous at first; that stage, however, doesn't last long. Part of adapting to an existence as a prostitute entails "protective denial," tamping down feelings, becoming numb, explains Sher (2011). For this reason, women and girls at the halfway house go to weekly Prostitutes Anonymous meetings, to learn how to face their reality, to learn to feel again. At the National Runaway Switchboard (NRS), many children cry out for someone to rescue them, but when they turn to people from their past, their pleas often fall on deaf ears. However, there are groups that do what they can to be available around the clock for the children on the street.

Sher (2011) says the phones ring incessantly at these switchboards, that runaway kids who end up on the street these days are getting younger and that the stretches of time they spend on the street are getting longer. Jennifer DiNicola, call center manager of the NRS, describes these children as afraid, in trouble, and traumatized.

The "darkness" that accompanies human trafficking is a good example of how projective identification can affect victims: negative feelings are spewed onto recipients, leaving them with toxic, bad feelings. The men who profit from the bodies they sell rid themselves of hostile emotions about sexuality (perhaps including thoughts of their own mothers and sisters) onto the girls in their power. Unconsciously the minds of these men may hold haunting strands of feeling, but consciously, having projected their evil thoughts onto the girls, they are pleased with themselves. They are, after all, "The Men" who make it all happen, and tend to reward themselves with lives of excess. On the other hand, they must constantly monitor the "property" they have commandeered and traumatized, making sure the women continue to accept their status as pawns with no dignity and no rights, a state induced and maintained by drugs or a loss of will.

Many girls, given their nightly repeated activities, readily accept as the truth what their pimps say: they are the scum of the earth. This is an example of how all-consuming projective identification can be and how it can erode one's sense of worth as a human being.

Internationally, human trafficking—although not exclusively for sexual purposes—is an illicit commerce right behind trafficking in drugs and weapons; its value is estimated at $150 billion annually (Konrad & Trapp, 2017). Wherever economies are struggling and families are large—from Southeast Asia to the Balkan states—merchants buy or kidnap children, subject them to a host of abuses, and then sell them to wealthier countries. Initially these human merchants may approach families with what sound like legitimate opportunities for a better life: employment or modeling, adoption, even marriage. These potential jobs or marriages are, of course, always in wealthier or better-developed countries. Parents may be won over by what sounds like a good future for their child—or they may be eager to transact, especially if the child is a girl, a future strain on their limited income. Some traffickers might persuade themselves that everyone is benefiting, including their captives, who will now get better "room and board." Most, however, are simply greedy (Drash, 2011).

Sher (2011) depicts child prostitutes as the orphans of our nation's justice system. While they tend to be disregarded, invisible, when they do have a run-in with law enforcement they are apt to be mistreated, arrested, and jailed while their pimps and customers, for the most part, go unpunished.

References

Dallaire, R. (2003). *Shake hands with the devil: The failure of humanity in Rwanda.* New York, NY: Carroll & Graf Publishers.
Des Forges, A. L. (1999). *Leave none to tell the story: Genocide in Rwanda* (Vol. 3169, No. 189). New York, NY: Human Rights Watch.
Drash, W. (2011). The CNN freedom project: Ending modern-day slavery. CNN.com.
Ferguson, J. (2017, May 3). How rape is used as a weapon in South Sudan's war. *PBS News Hour.*
Fullerton, D. (2011). Origins, Hutu and Tutsi. Rwandanstories.org.
Incredible stories of forgiveness—Portraits of reconciliation. (2014). Galactic Free Press.
Johnson, D. (2002, January 25). The red army's WWII horror: Orgy of rape worse than thought. Rense.com.
King, C. I. (2016, January 15). Washington DC's serious sex-trafficking problem. *The Washington Post.*
Konrad, R. & Trapp, A. C. (2017, July 29). Data science can help us fight human trafficking. *PBS News Hour.*
Kristof, N. (2017, January 12). A website peddling girls for sex. *The New York Times.*
Neill, K. G. (2000). Duty, honor, rape: Sexual assault against women during war. *Journal of International Women's Studies, 2*(1), 43–51.
Noble, A. (2013, December 5). D.C. police officer linked to prostitution ring. *The Washington Times.*
Outreach programme on the Rwanda Genocide and the United Nations. UN.org.
Petrova, D. (2016a, June 10). Sex trafficking in Brooklyn demands visibility, accountability: "Everyone knows that the police won't do anything." Salon.com.
Petrova, D. (2016b, January 17). The scourge of human trafficking: It's not just other countries' problem. Salon.com.
Resource Information Center. (2001, August 14). Information on the role of the Interhamwe militia and the use of roadblocks during the 1994 Rwandan genocide. Refworld.org.
Rizvanolli, I., Bean, L. & Farnsworth, N. (2005). Kosovar civil society report to the United Nations on violence against women in Kosovo. UN.org.
Robbins, R. H. (1999, repr. 2002). *Global problems and the culture of capitalism.* Boston, MA: Allyn & Bacon.
Sher, J. (2011). *Somebody's daughter: The hidden story of America's prostituted children and the battle to save them.* Chicago, IL: Chicago Review Press.
Smyth, F. (1996). Rwanda's butchers: The Interahamwe and former Rwandan army. *Jane's Intelligence Review,* Special Report No. 13.
Uvin, P. (2009). *Life after violence: A people's story of Burundi.* London and New York, NY: Zed Books.
Wilson, M. (2017, January 15). Runaway teenager slowly reveals tale of horrors while away. *The New York Times.*

PART IV

Mechanisms that reverse the damage

Mentalization and reparative leadership as antidotes to projective identification

10

ATTACHMENT, ATTACHMENT TRAUMA, AND MENTALIZATION

Key components that affect the development of the self and the formation of group identity

Attachment

A key to happiness and fulfillment in life emanates from a secure attachment with another person or persons. We all grow and thrive based on this premise. We also come to know about our external as well as our internal world from others; new information we acquire has already been known by someone else. Wolfgang Prinz (2012) captures this idea and elaborates on it in his explanation of social mirroring, a phenomenon he says:

> ...can help with building architectures for experience from preexisting architectures for behavioral performance ... Minds are open in two senses: One is that they are made and molded in and through the mirror of others, thus designing themselves after others. The other is that they're open and highly susceptible to any knowledge they may attain concerning others' acting, thinking, and knowing.
>
> *(Prinz, 2012, p. xvi)*

If a person is lucky enough to be securely attached to a caregiver as an infant through the process of mirroring, the world starts out as a safe place. If one doesn't have this good fortune, life can be bleak. Paradoxically, unlike material inheritance, early attachment is intangible, and can only be judged from emotions and behavior later in life.

According to the seminal research findings of Mary Ainsworth (1969) and John Bowlby (1969) babies seek attachment from birth. It serves as a major motivational force that is as important as other instinctual drives throughout life. As Bowlby (1969) put it, it is important "from cradle to grave." Hence, all babies need a secure bond and an emotional connection with a primary caregiver in which the child can grow, prosper, and "bloom" in a safe environment, since the optimum way a baby develops is through exploration. In the shadow of the securely attached mother, father or other appropriate person, a child can learn about his or her new fascinating surroundings. Enchanting discoveries can be made as long as the safe person is present, which the child checks to verify from time to time. Whether the area is filled with bright new unusual shapes, old cardboard boxes, or alluring toys waiting to be found, the baby or toddler who is psychologically secure can encounter, explore, and thrive in his or her world.

Attachment trauma

When the feeling of safety is in question, however—due to some severe threat—the happy picture of normal development changes. If neglect or abuse occurs, physical and psychological safety no longer exist. When the safe person can no longer protect the child, trust is broken. The child recipient of abuse becomes filled with despair because he or she has been neglected, abused, or even brutalized in attacks that cut off access to his or her sense of self. Such acts against children usually bring about a major change, one that results in an attachment trauma, a state of being akin to the death of the psyche.

Along with causing physical or emotional pain, attachment trauma strips away a person's dignity, damaging to an adult and even more destructive for a child. It also frequently induces a feeling of shame that is accompanied by a wish to hide. When this occurs, the recipient of the abuse does not think she or he did something bad, but that he or she *is* bad, which makes connections with another person very difficult. Thus, an attachment trauma frequently robs the victim of his or her ability to have meaningful long-term relationships because he or she decouples his or her mind from the minds of other people and reverts to less organized and more fragmented states of the self. Hence, much is lost in terms of having meaningful connections with other people (Fonagy & Bateman, 2006).

Meanwhile, the perpetrator of pain and abuse can expel his or her own sense of "badness" onto the helpless child (or adolescent or adult) because he or she cannot tolerate this aspect of the self. What cannot be tolerated by one person is projected onto another, which leads to massive projective identification. Mature relationships become less and less possible. Thus, attachment trauma is tantamount to destruction of personality.

Moreover, when a person who was not securely attached to a caregiver as a child is abused, his or her experience of trauma is likely to be far worse than that of a securely attached person. However, attachment style is not the only important factor to take into account. In addition to how well attached a person was to his or her primary caregiver, *who* abused the person is also very important (Bohleber, 2010).

Whether or not the event or situation has a traumatic effect depends on whether an intensive relationship existed between the child and the traumatogenic character. This view of the way in which childhood traumata occur proved to be very fruitful in terms of research and therapy. As confirmed by one longitudinal study (Steele, 1994), in cases of maltreatment or abuse it is not primarily the physical injury of the child that causes the trauma disorder; the most pathogenic element is that of being mistreated or abused by the person whom one needs for actual protection and care (Bohleber, 2010).

C. Fred Alford (2016) adds to the discussion about the effects of abuse with his description of the "inner other," that internal voice or sense of ourselves with whom we have a type of silent dialogue. He indicates that no matter when it occurs, severe trauma shuts down self-awareness so that victims have little sense of themselves. They cannot navigate comfortably in this world without their "inner other." In addition to the loss of possibility for a secure attachment to another person, the sense of self is out of reach. Alford (2016), however, offers hope by suggesting that with the recovery of the "inner other" to provide guidance through internal communication, in fact to permit a rich mentalization, one can make it through life.

The "inner other" is not to be confused with the superego, since it is not harsh or punitive. It is more like an internal compass; it helps us decide what we want in life and how we can obtain it, from simple preferences to major decisions. To me, the inner other is that sense of yourself that helps you decide whether you want to play tennis or visit someone in an assisted-living facility. Without this mechanism it is as if we know neither where we are going nor how to get there. It would be like driving a car without being able to see. This concept reminded me of something I have sometimes said to patients: "You aren't ever really alone. You always have yourself as company. That's why it's important to take care of yourself and like yourself." I have felt this inner consciousness myself, and it has been very comforting.

But for a person who has been traumatized—whether by wartime encounters, by sexual abuse, or some other psychic suffering—it is extremely difficult to mentalize this sense of one's "inner other" because someone else's "truth" has been forced upon him or her, erasing all of his or her own control and personal power. Quite often he or she has been forced to watch, even participate in, all kinds of heinous acts. Frequently the traumatized person has been mentally wounded, raped, or brutally deprived of dignity and selfhood. What kind of therapy do such people need to help recover, to restore self-respect and a sense of well-being?

Successful attachment: a personal view

People inherit all kinds of things from their parents: wealth, yachts, or the old family home. However, from a psychoanalytic point of view, the best legacy is an intangible sense of who they are as people—a secure attachment from their earliest days on earth. Paradoxically, unlike material inheritance, early attachment cannot be remembered, but only judged (or when necessary, diagnosed) from emotions and behavior later in life. In my case, I have known for years how fortunate I was in the secure base my parents gave me.

In the slow dance between holding and gradually letting go, my parents seemed to know the right steps in their bones. In my earliest memories, it is clear to me that they were there; yet I also knew I could wander and explore the world around me, as well as my internal world, without their over-protectiveness. Among my earliest memories of childhood I remember naps: a special time of day alone with my mother, who read to me from a green fairy-tale book in a warm, cuddly exchange. I remember feeling so peaceful and safe as she read each story in the book many times; "The Princess and the Pea" is one I remember, perhaps because I felt like a princess. A longer, more exotic choice was *Hans Brinker, or the Silver Skates*. I asked a lot of questions until my eyes slowly closed as I fell asleep by my mother's side. When I think of those times now, I recall how soothing her voice was.

We lived on several islands in the Florida Keys as I was growing up. In Marathon I remember playing in the sand with a silver ladle as my mother sat in a chair nearby and watched me collect shells and other special treasures that I placed in my bucket. I have no idea why I was playing with her piece of silver, but I remember really liking it. When I was older she gave it to me; when I look at it now, it takes me back to those lovely, carefree days in the sun.

My father—a wandering spirit who moved us from a 180-foot schooner to Islamorada and then to Marathon—was also part of my sense of security. Both of them often took me to a dock near our house, where my father taught me to fish. I remember with delight those times when I pulled up my pole and had a fish on the line. A photo of a three- or four-year-old, grinning ear-to-ear and proudly hoisting her catch toward the camera, is a souvenir of those days. When I was with them together, or with one or the other, I felt so safe and protected. Since I had no siblings, they had plenty of time to spend with me, and they apparently enjoyed it. Later, when my gregarious father settled down to run Ralph's Restaurant, my mother and I joined him.

My mother, who was a homemaker until I was a teenager, was the primary caregiver, handling many of the day-to-day tasks of raising a child. Always ready to talk, always available to share my joy as well as my pain, she was my go-to person whether I was happy or hurt. She also set limits. If I wanted something she thought I wasn't yet old enough for, it was understood that the wish itself was perfectly okay; however, that didn't mean I could have the desired object. Her message was that anticipation was a good thing; there was value in waiting until one was ready. Trusting her judgment, I never felt deprived. As I grew up, I came to appreciate her wisdom.

Another important quality that I learned through watching my mother is patience. She never got angry at me for mistakes, crazy impulses, or for not knowing something. Her position was that together we could finish whatever frustrating task had to be done. When as a second grader I "volunteered" her time to make a fancy Valentine's Day box overnight, she took it in stride and elaborately decorated a box that I was proud to take to school the next day. My mother never infringed on my growth or development either; she nudged but never pushed me. I remember once not wanting to go into a Saturday catechism class because I was late. I'm sure it frustrated her, but she didn't make me go into the class. Knowing I was embarrassed and upset, she talked to me about my feelings, gave me a kiss on my forehead, and said she knew how difficult it was to feel embarrassed. Then she remarked that there was always next week. Equally important to secure attachment, I was never humiliated or shamed by either parent when I didn't do what I was supposed to do. Instead, they talked to me about why I should or shouldn't do it, instilling a regard for honesty and openness.

My parents never tried to impose their opinions on me, but rather encouraged me to have my own views. During the Kennedy/Nixon presidential race of 1960, as a young fan of politics I was for John Kennedy, while my father was a Nixon man. He encouraged me to challenge his views and to stand up for what mattered to me. Like the results of the Clinton/Trump presidential race, the tally was not certain. When I went to bed, it looked as though Nixon had won. I got up the next day without knowing what had happened in the wee hours of the morning. In the kitchen I met my father, who had in front of him a ten-dollar bill and a glass of orange juice for me. He indicated that we were going to have a new president in the White House—President-elect Kennedy— and said I had done a good job presenting my ideas. Elated, I gave him a hug and ran to find the paper. I was never taught to think as my parents thought; the world was mine to discover.

Eventual independence was a goal, beginning with the time, at about age seven, when I was first allowed to ride my bicycle to the variety store a half-mile away to buy a $2 toy; I felt so grown-up! And when it was time for me to leave for college at 17, with tears in our eyes we packed the car, and my parents watched as I drove off. I knew it was hard for them, but my excitement about my new life eased their feelings of sadness. My leaving the Keys to pursue my dreams was never a question. My mother knew that children are not objects one keeps, but gifts one receives for a time but not forever.

What's the link between mentalization and attachment?

Attachment and mentalizing are inextricably connected. Where there is a secure attachment, the capacity to explore the mind of another person is possible. Specifically, when a child has a secure attachment, the attachment figure is interested in the child's mind, making it safe for the child to explore the mind of that attachment figure. Hence, babies begin to feel safe when they are known to the caregiver.

When this occurs, the child is able to explore the mind of the other. As noted earlier, this is how he or she learns about the self—through the eyes of the caregiver who has taken the other in and made meaning of this person, who can then experience himself or herself based on the interpretation of the caregiver. Taken together, attachment and mentalization could be thought of as an antidote to projective identification. As a person in the paranoid-schizoid position begins to experience the other, he or she moves toward the depressive position. When this occurs, a person starts to see another as a whole object; there is an opportunity to view oneself as an individual person as well. One can begin to realize that he or she has a mind and the other person does as well. At this point there aren't fantasies of fusion or a need to cling to a sense of being part of the other person.

The link between attachment and mentalizing is clear. Attachment contexts provide the ideal conditions for fostering mentalizing. Secure attachment relationships, where attachment figures are interested in the child's mind and the child is safe to explore the mind of the attachment figure (Fonagy, Campbell & Luyten, 2014), allow the child or infant to explore other subjectivities, including that of his/her caregiver. Finding him- or herself accurately represented in the mind of the caregiver as a thinking and feeling intentional being ensures that the infant's own capacities for mentalizing will develop well (Fonagy, Gergely, Jurist & Target, 2002).

As it relates to the process of psychoanalytic thinking, mentalization was not the word used by interpersonalists. However, the essence of what they were trying to convey was similar as indicated by Clara Thompson in 1956. She said that she and some of her colleagues including Sullivan and Fromm-Reichman had been working much like Ferenczi with good results. She stressed this new technique included more frankness about the analyst's role (Thompson, 1956). In essence, the interpersonalists were interested in two people working together to understand the mind of the other person.

Mentalization as the foundation for thinking

When thinking about the atrocities that have taken place in our modern world, it is important to consider what can be done to ameliorate misery. How can we help victims and even perpetrators of terrorism and trauma—all of them—to reduce their fearful projections and become empathic? As I have suggested, one way is by helping people develop the capacity to mentalize in a variety of ways after they have experienced a more optimum and secure attachment with another person (or a safe group) who understands their point of view.

This process sounds straightforward but it is more complex than meets the eye. For one thing, the term itself is unfamiliar to many people, even to psychotherapists. It is actually a concept that is quite old, but was not widely used in the U.S. or England until Peter Fonagy, Jon Allen and their colleagues began to write about it approximately 25 years ago (Freeman, 2016). The word defines an ability that everyone must have or acquire in order to participate effectively in relationships with other people. Fundamentally, it means being able to recognize one's feelings and thoughts and, just as important, to recognize, understand,

and accept that others have their own different thoughts, ideas, and feelings. If this process is not developed and nurtured in childhood, it must be learned in adulthood in order to have meaningful personal, social, civic, and professional encounters with others. To allow another person to become who he or she is as an individual is essential. According to Jon Allen in his book *Plain Old Therapy* (2012), many theorists and therapists incorporate the techniques of learning to mentalize into their treatment without using the name.

The idea seems simple enough, and well-adapted people have little difficulty with it. As Fonagy and his colleagues (2002) have said, mentalizing is a form of perceiving and interpreting human behavior in terms of intentional mental states—e.g. needs, desires, feelings, beliefs, goals, purposes, and reasons (Fonagy, Gergely, Jurist & Target, 2002). Also, since the ability to mentalize is important in all situations where communication is involved, it is an essential capacity. It is recognized in many fields other than that of psychoanalytic theory, perhaps especially in philosophy, where epistemologists take up the problem of thinking about the minds of others (Goodnight, 2013).

In discussions within groups where members are tenaciously affixed to opposing ideas, there is often little mentalizing going on. Take, for example, the primary Presidential election campaign of 2015–16. Even among themselves, the Republican candidates were unable to understand the viewpoint of the other. When on the campaign trail or during debates, they did not say that there might be different ways to think about what would be best for the country. Little or no understanding of another's point of view emerged. This tone was set as early as the announcement of each candidate's decision to run. If, in their heated debates, even one candidate had said something like, "Senator, I understand your points, and you have every right to think that you know the best way to proceed. I happen to have a different idea about slowing down global warming," it might have made a difference. That would have been an example of having the capacity to mentalize. However, this ability did not seem to be exhibited by the debaters. Instead, for the most part it seemed to be absent. Ideas were projected onto voters as if each opinion were a fact. Hence, the candidates were operating in a paranoid-schizoid position. They weren't considering the thoughts of others and were stuck.

While it didn't happen for the 2016 Presidential candidates, some people do emerge from Klein's (1946) paranoid-schizoid position of projection. When aggression and other unbearable feelings are modulated, modified, or made tolerable in some manner, the way of experiencing the self and others can shift. Movement or growth occurs. This second state or way of relating to the world, Klein's (1946) depressive position, creates an atmosphere wherein hostile feelings can be understood, reclaimed, or "taken back." They no longer must be projected but can be experienced as belonging to the self. Others are now thought of as whole people, with various qualities and characteristics. Some of the qualities exhibited by other people may be appreciated and some not, but the person in the depressive position realizes that good and bad characteristics can coexist in the same person, without one part having to be eradicated or disavowed. In this position, opportunities for mourning, repair, and learning from past experience become possible. Rational thinking is also restored. With the help of another or others, the process of change occurs in the context of a relational world wherein one's initial raw aggression is modified and made bearable. This is what must occur for someone to move from one position to the other. Hope becomes possible when raw aggression and aggressive tendencies are modified, a change that is a form of identification with the essence of the other (Klein, 1946).

While different terms have been used to describe how change of this type comes about, one most notably was described by a follower of Klein's, Wilfred Bion (1962). He called it "containment" and the "alpha function." In this process, aggression in all its forms is transformed and made tolerable and acceptable to the person who projected the confusing and difficult-to-manage feelings and thoughts in the first place.

Applying this concept to everyday life

I began to theorize about this important concept in some depth in 2008 as I prepared a paper for presentation. While drafting "Taking Back Projections: The Hope and Despair in Projective Identification," I came to realize that recipients of negative projections might benefit if mentalization became part of their worldview. There is obvious pain and despair in the type of projection associated with trauma, mostly for the recipient, but I began to see how hope could arise out of the process as well. Mentalization, I hypothesized, could be an important part of helping a patient to grow or recover if projections were "taken back." It is a reason to hope.

The key to mentalization: attachment

But how are the qualities and skills that help one mentalize acquired? Contemporary scholars such as Fonagy and Bateman (2008) and Fonagy and Allen (2006) have done thoughtful research to try to discover how mentalization develops, and how it can be taught. They believe it is through identification with others that this state of mind comes into being. Hence, as many experts in development, attachment, and mentalization have said, the care for one's children is imperative, particularly the way they are cared for by their parents early in life (Sroufe, 2005).

If young children are to develop into adults who are intrapsychically healthy, they need a caregiver to help them maintain safe inner worlds by metabolizing their anxieties and fears, making them more palatable. Growing children can gradually take responsibility for and tolerate aspects of their lives that they initially projected outward because they could not bear overwhelming and intolerable feelings. In short, babies who are securely attached to their primary caretaker are much more likely to learn how to mentalize, as long as that caretaker is successful at mentalizing.

Seeing "the child as an intentional being"—one with a mind of his or her own—is the caregiver's great gift to the developing infant and permits that child gradually to perceive the caregiver as a separate person with a life of his or her own as well. Such children are far less likely to experience hostile emotions that go unsmoothed and unresolved and are less likely to construct a "not-me" sense of self against which they will later need to build unconscious defenses.

There is also growing evidence that mentalization is related to certain aspects of neuroscience that focus on listening theory. In his 2013 paper, "Mirroring, Mentalizing, and the Social Neurosciences," Robert Spunt discusses the important connection between listening and mentalizing from a neuroscience perspective, including the need for active interpretation as well as gleaning what is said and not said in verbal as well as non-verbal communication.

Such theorization has strong implications for mentalization in the therapeutic dyad, as well as in intimate and personal relationships that require deep acceptance of the humanity of the other. In fact, mentalization reflects, albeit through a different prism, the therapeutic relationships that Sándor Ferenczi, Clara Thompson, and to some extent Harry Stack Sullivan were trying to develop. The idea of two people (the analyst and the patient) working together through understanding each other's minds was the essence of these interpersonalists' work. In the 21st century, following the widespread adoption of relationalist theory, I share Jon Allen's (2012) view that it is useful (I would say essential) to keep the concept of mentalizing in mind, as well as the ideas inherent in attachment theory, as we set about to work with patients in psychotherapy and, I would add, psychoanalysis.

Mentalizing and non-mentalizing

In many situations in life, projective identification, the "taking back" of projections and aspects of attachment and mentalization can be observed when examining exchanges between people, e.g., when considering exchanges between babies and mothers. Take the jealous toddler with the teething little brother. If she is picked up, talked to, and held by a patient mother who soothes and comforts her, demonstrating feelings of love and inclusion, what seemed unbearable becomes tolerable. The child's world is okay again. She settles down, stops crying, and reengages with her surroundings. Though observers often do not know exactly what initially troubled the young child, the intensity of the distress makes clear that the feelings involved in the episode were difficult—more than the child could handle alone. Over time, as the mother handles additional states of intense anger and projected aggression in a similar way, the toddler eventually takes in and identifies with the mother's attitude and makes it her own. She comes to know through experience that the new baby will not totally replace her, that there is room for both, and that love from the mother is still available. She learns how to integrate her baby brother into her life by taking in transformed aggression and using it more productively. Eventually, patience develops.

A similar, more mature process can occur in adulthood. An example is the case of John, a patient who projected onto both his former lover and then onto me (I originally described this patient in Chapter 1).

As I was able to mentally take in and bear John's rage and emotional pain, and thereafter "give it back" to him in a more palatable form through interpretation, he eventually came to understand how the feelings he was attributing to me were actually feelings he had that he could not tolerate. He eventually grasped that he wished to get rid of me as a therapist because I reminded him of his unbearable experience with Alison, the former lover; getting rid of me in his fantasy was a way to get rid of her. John planned to leave me as she had left him, so that I/Alison would understand the intensity of his pain. Eventually we came to understand together that he needed me to hold onto and tolerate the aggression he felt because it frightened him so much. He was afraid of his anger, hatred, and rage toward Alison for deceiving and then leaving him.

Once John began to recognize his own emotions accurately, his wife, Susan, became much more real to him. She became a person he had once loved, even still loved, but also someone who was not perfect. As he began taking responsibility for his contribution to the situation while dealing with the loss of his fantasy woman, he also began to see his wife as someone with whom he could have a real relationship. As John acknowledged the damage he had done to Susan and their marriage, he began to mourn what had been lost between them. Thereafter he was able to feel grief and sadness over his actions and to apologize for his affair, thus allowing the process of reparation to begin. Only through acknowledgement of his transgressions was he able to experience true sorrow, which led to repair.

As John moved from the paranoid-schizoid to the depressive position, self-knowledge and the capacity to think rationally were restored to him as well. He was able to know his own pain better, and to bear it more easily. He took in and made his own the experience he gained from our work together as he mourned the loss of what could not be. As he began the process of repair with his wife as well as with me, both of us became whole people to him—with negative as well as positive attributes.

When we are most vulnerable, we all have the potential for moments of extreme anger and projection. When we reconstitute ourselves, however (because we have learned to do so from someone else at an earlier time, or because we have effective therapy), we move to the more integrated depressive position wherein we can experience all aspects of the people that we meet, and accept them for who they are. In this position we grapple with the human condition that includes suffering, pain, sadness, and sorrow. These emotions help us to become more authentic beings as we change and grow.

References

Ainsworth, M. D. S. (1969). Object relations, dependency and attachment: A theoretical review of the infant-mother relationship. *Child Development*, *40*(4), 969–1025.

Alford, C. F. (2016). *Trauma, culture, and PTSD*. New York, NY: Palgrave Macmillan.
Allen, J. G. (2012). *Restoring mentalizing in attachment relationships: Treating trauma with plain old therapy*. Washington, DC: American Psychiatric Association Publishing.
Allen, J. G., Fonagy, P. & Bateman, A. W. (2008). *Mentalizing in clinical practice.* Washington, DC: American Psychiatric Association Publishing.
Bion, W. (1962). A theory of thinking. In *Second thoughts: Selected papers on psychoanalysis*, pp. 110–119. New York, NY: Jason Aronson.
Bohleber, W. (2010). *Destructiveness, intersubjectivity, and trauma: The identity crisis of modern psychoanalysis*. London: Karnac Books.
Bowlby, J. (1969). *Attachment and loss*. New York, NY: Basic Books.
Fonagy, P. & Allen, J. G. (2006). *Handbook of mentalization-based treatment*. New York, NY: John Wiley & Sons.
Fonagy, P. & Bateman, A. W. (2006). Mechanisms of change in mentalization-based treatment of BPD. *Journal of Clinical Psychology, 62*(4), 411–430.
Fonagy, P. & Bateman, A. (2008). The development of borderline personality disorder—A mentalizing model. *Journal of Personality Disorders, 22*, 4–21.
Fonagy, P., Gergely, G., Jurist, E. L. & Target, M. (Eds.). (2002). *Affect regulation, mentalization, and the development of the self*. New York, NY: Other Press.
Fonagy, P., Luyten, P., Campbell, C. (2014, December). Epistemic trust, psychopathology, and the great psychotherapy debate. *Society for the Advancement of Psychotherapy*. Society for Psychotherapy.
Freeman, C. (2016). What is mentalizing? An overview. *British Journal of Psychotherapy, 32*(2), 189–201.
Goodnight, G. T. (2013). The virtues of reason and the problem of other minds: Reflections on argumentation in a new century. OSSA Conference Archive, 2, pp. 1–17.
Klein, M. (1946). Notes on some schizoid mechanisms. *International Journal of Psycho-Analysis, 27*, 99–110.
Prinz, W. (2012). *Open minds: The social making of agency and intentionality*. Cambridge, MA: MIT Press.
Spunt, R. P. (2013). Mirroring, mentalizing, and the social neuroscience of listening. *International Journal of Listening, 27*(2), 61–72.
Sroufe, L. (2005) Attachment and development: A prospective, longitudinal study from birth to adulthood. *Attachment and Human Development, 4*, 349–367.
Steele, B. F. (1994). Psychoanalysis and the maltreatment of children. *Journal of the American Psychoanalytic Association, 42*, 1001–1025.
Thompson, C. M. (1956). The role of the analyst's personality in therapy. In M. R. Green (Ed.), *Interpersonal Psychoanalysis*, New York: Basic Books.

11
REPARATIVE LEADERSHIP AS A WAY TO HELP GROUPS
Reconciliation in Rwanda as an example of hope

As discussed previously, while it is possible to help an individual, one might justifiably wonder how this type of change could ever be attempted when considering terrorism or any other massively projected action against a group of people. In this chapter the focus is placed on how animosity in groups can be decreased or eliminated through repair. I believe this can be done by applying the principles inherent in the integrative process of mentalization to the isolation of projective identification. If we can find a way to metabolize aggression on a large scale, if we can persuade groups to "own" their aggression, mourn what is lost or cannot be, then we can collectively work toward repairing misunderstandings and accepting the uniqueness—and the rights—of others. In so doing, the possibility of hope is created by developing or restoring connections with another person or other people.

By considering essential components of projective identification and mentalization, cultural leaders, diplomats, and those in charge of implementing change on a grand scale can find a way to help people metabolize aggression on a large scale. Thereafter, when group members can be persuaded to "own" their aggression and mourn what is lost or cannot be, hostile forces can collectively work toward repairing misunderstandings while accepting the uniqueness, the humanity—and the rights—of others.

C. Fred Alford (1989) has grappled with aspects of Klein's thinking to address key problems raised by the Frankfurt School that he referred to as the "four Rs." "Remembrance of those who suffered; Reparation for their loss; Reformation of reason; and Reconciliation with nature" (Alford, 1989, p. 170).

Notice that "remorse" does not appear on Alford's (1989) list of key goals. Pointless emotions, even expressions of regret and apologies for past actions, are not the issue; rather, a resolute forward vision and a determination to act in new ways in light of the past are what make all the difference. In essence, Alford

(1989) believes that because Klein (1946) focused on the "need" for suffering as she moved beyond Freud's (1920) pleasure principle, she developed the possibility of hope through an understanding and tolerance of emotional pain. In other words, change is possible if one embarks on those four Rs while keeping in mind the suffering of others past and present, and making amends for one's own errors in a thoughtful manner as one gradually reconciles with all aspects of what it means to be human.

The right leaders

Alford (1989) adds another dimension as he applies Kleinian theory to groups in what he calls "reparative leadership" (pp. 89–90). He claims that responsible political leaders will recognize that the public is often scared to death of its own aggressive urges, as well as those of the enemy. Responsible leaders will therefore not exaggerate the "goodness" of their own group and the "badness" of the other. Referring to the opposition as an "evil empire" only encourages divisiveness and projection.

Who is the reparative leader? Alford (1989) asks. One for whom the opposition, no matter how intensely fought, remains part of a moral or ethical whole to which all people belong. As part of the whole, the opposition partakes of the good; it is not simply the evil other. Such a leader also recognizes that his own group's claim to goodness is incomplete. The reparative leader does not protect either his leadership or the unity of his group by demonizing others. Rather, his or her leadership is based upon the ability to interpret the group's moral tradition in such a way that it includes the opponent—without, however, utterly remaking the opponent and denying that person or group's otherness. The last clause is important, adds Alford (1989); Mahatma Gandhi, Martin Luther King, and Nelson Mandela readily come to his mind as genuine reparative leaders (p. 90). In brief, Alford tell us that reparative leaders exhibit effective behavior, consistent with the depressive position, when they metabolize aggression and anxiety on behalf of the people they govern. Through the process of mentalization, they hold in mind the positive attributes of "enemies" without demanding that they give up their identities.

Real roadblocks to progress remain. Alford (1989) suggests that post-traumatic stress disorder is not the medical condition that psychiatry assumes, but a cultural and political phenomenon. His evidence: events that have traumatic effects on people in one culture do not necessarily in another, depending significantly on available traditions and community institutions for group support. For example, few Sri Lankans were "traumatized" in the Western sense by the 2004 tsunami. Similarly, I think, "terrorism" has become a political diagnosis or cultural construct. The transition began when, after 9/11, George W. Bush declared a "war on terror" (Address to a Joint Session of Congress, 2001, September 20) as if armies could defeat a centuries-old political tactic. The next step was growing acceptance, on the American political scene, of demonizing all Muslims as terrorists. Today, whenever someone brings out a gun and shoots in a public place—as happened near Seattle in late 2016, in Montreal in early 2017, in pre-election Paris in late April 2017—he is likely to be described as having suspiciously dark "foreign" features.

Eventually the media learn that he may be mentally troubled and has no Arab ancestry, but is a "home-grown" terrorist—then their reports seem to convey an air of disappointment. From my perspective, projective identification by radical jihadists of their own humiliation and hatred onto the West has, in turn, led some Europeans and Americans to demonize Muslims generally. This equating of "Muslim" with "terrorist," disregarding all individuality for ethnic characteristics, promptly galvanized the Trump administration and its supporters. It is projection on a massive, international scale. I believe acts of terror occur because, like energy in the physical world, aggression cannot be destroyed, only modified, contained, understood, or dealt with productively within groups of people. When it is not modified by some form of conversation, it is most often projected outward and affects others—sometimes mildly, sometimes moderately, and sometimes in the most devastating and destructive ways.

I have talked about the theoretical aspect of change by considering Kleinian theory, and suggested, along with Alford (1989), that powerful, self-aware leaders can make a difference, but a major question remains regarding opportunities for change. In our complex world, how can private individuals have any impact on a broad basis? A partial answer may be found by combining the four Rs with the skills inherent in mentalizing. If we have the conviction that we can teach individuals and the members of a group of any size, large or small, then the route to success is imaginable, perhaps even visible on the horizon on a clear day.

This is in conjunction with the components of attachment and mentalization that apply to groups. One important consideration that must be addressed when helping people on a large or small scale is how the projected anxiety is handled by those attempting to assist others, since traumatized people are often immobilized. In order to help others who are lost in a projective-identification process, one must be able to experience intense projections as a way of communicating. In so doing, potential helpers must "take on" and metabolize massive projections without becoming destabilized. While this is crucially important, it is not something that is always known by people in the helping professions.

The way in which Rwandans came together after the 1994 genocide is an illustration of how a fractured group can heal; being able to put themselves in the other's shoes set the tone for reconciliation. As this occurred, people in both tribes began to understand themselves and their motivation more clearly as well as understanding their former enemy's previous position (Al Jazeera, 2015).

Reconciliation in Rwanda: an example of group mentalization

A version of groups learning to mentalize occurred in Rwanda in the reconciliation between Hutus and Tutsis after the genocide of 1994 (Rwanda is discussed in Chapter 10). The results tell us that healing can occur, though not necessarily how it happens. What occurred appears to be akin to Alford's "reparative leadership." Rwandans have managed to build a successful economy and, apparently, society, together. How did it come about? There are various hypotheses, beginning with the powerful leadership of Paul Kagame, transformed from Tutsi rebel commander to national civilian president. Although I have only secondhand knowledge from Roméo Dallaire and others (2003) on the scene, I still speculate that Kagame had, or has developed, a remarkable capacity for mentalization of others' views and has achieved the Kleinian depressive position.

These preliminary steps allowed many Rwandans to develop the capacity to mentalize. One guiding principle that contributed to the success of bringing Tutsis and Hutus together is public recognition of hard truths (Sebaranzi, 2009). What also led to peace in Rwanda was the country's use of the model of the South African Commission on Truth and Reconciliation, designed by Nelson Mandela and Desmond Tutu, in which Afrikaners admitted to their cruel actions in front of black Africans (ADST, 2015). In Rwanda, Hutus and Tutsis have been forgiven, as long as they owned up to what they did (with what level of sincerity we cannot know). When projections of inhumanity are "taken back," when some new understanding of the previously demonized can develop, reconciliation is possible. This step is essential when seeking broad and genuine buy-in to put an end to major conflicts, and not mere truce or armistice.

After the genocide, Paul Kagame was instrumental in helping people come together while working toward a common goal. One way this happened in Rwanda was by reinstituting *umuganda*, a process that involves people gathering and then working together to accomplish a specific, shared task. This concept allowed people to heal (Sigri, 2010). In 2017, a similar effort was planned for Colombia in an effort to reintegrate FARC narco-guerrillas and at least two rebel groups. Due to his effort to reunite these groups, President Juan Manuel Santos was awarded the Noble Peace Prize in 2016 (Casey, 2016).

On another level, important healing can happen by simple acts of working together across boundaries. This was the contribution of Rwandan women, Hutu and Tutsi, who had rarely been killers but often victims. While tolerating their intrapsychic pain, they seem to have had the mindset that they could grieve for many years or move on. They chose the latter. Drawing upon deep shared roots, they turned to the craft of Rwandan basketry, created workshops, revived traditional designs, and marketed their products as widely as possible (Seymour, 2007). When commitment to a common project was maintained by all concerned, real social advancement occurred.

The results of focusing on the future while not totally forgetting the past seem to have led to a remarkable outcome. While they did not create a utopian state, the transformation in Rwanda since the 1994 genocide is pretty amazing when one considers how many other places in the world have been warring psychologically if not engaged in actual combat for decades if not centuries.

It is nothing short of a miracle to see the changes in Rwanda since the civil war of 1994. For the Rwandan government to conceive of a way to help tribal divides dissipate was a monumental achievement in bringing about a holistic culture so that its people could become, first and foremost, "Rwandan." Now the idea of "Rwandan-ness" is proudly hailed by all. As each year of this successful experiment progresses, the history of those warring years among the Tutsi, Hutu, and Twa fades even further into the mist (Tumwebaze, 2015).

Ms. Odile Katese's contribution (Arlin, 2011) provided one of the many successful stories of overcoming past hostilities and hatred by bringing together a group of Tutsi and Hutu women to form Ingoma Nishya ("New Drum" or "New Kingdom"), a drumming troupe. This was notable for two reasons. The first one related to unity. Up to this point, Tutsi and Hutu women would not join any type of mutual cause. The second issue involved male versus female activities. Prior to Katese's initiative, drumming was the sole province of men. The troupe not only gave the women a forum for music; more importantly, it was a vehicle for healing for the women who had been raped and mutilated in battles between the Hutu and Tutsi.

To provide spaces where people could feel safe again, free of fear and hatred, in 2010, after meeting with women in New York who had created a successful organic ice cream store, Katese founded the first organic ice cream shop in the town of Butare. She named it Inzozi Nziza (Sweet Dreams). It is owned and operated by a cooperative consisting of all of the drummers from the troupe. After getting off to a slow start, the women persevered. They got an interview on a radio station with male drummers from Burundi that increased the visibility of their performing art as well as the sales in their ice cream shop (Yerman, 2012). This endeavor—putting together the drumming troupe and building the structure for the ice cream shop—highlights the idea that we can wait for others to step forward to do what is needed to make necessary changes, but at some point someone has to take charge by organizing a small group of people to inspire others to change.

To take an example far from Africa, indigenous women from the Molo tribe on Timor, an island in West Indonesia, banded together when the local government gave the go-ahead for marble extraction companies to mine on Mutis Mountain—the source of all the rivers on the island, and sacred to the Molo. When the clearing and digging began in 1996, Aleta Baun and three colleagues went from village to distant village, calling their people to remember that the mountain is their body, its rivers their blood, its forest their hair—and that its plants provide the dyes used in indigenous women's weaving, an important part of their economic and social lives. In 2006 some 100 women (the traditional landowners among the Molo) went to a quarry, formed their looms in a circle, and performed a silent "weaving occupation" for more than a year. They persisted (Merlino, 2014).

Rapid change between warring entities rarely happens so fast. More frequently than not, animosity and hatred between rival groups lasts for hundreds of years or more. Sadly, the Sunni–Shia ideological conflict over the authenticity of Muhammad's successor began shortly after the prophet died in the 6th century.

Another example of failed reconciliation is still occurring between the Turks and the Armenians. The genocide in Armenia that occurred more than 103 years ago is not being acknowledged by many people. It is still being denied by Turkey as well as by other countries that apparently do not want to get involved for fear of getting on the wrong side of the Turkish government. However, the events that occurred beginning on April 24, 1915 have not been forgotten by the Armenian people and their descendants (Klemack, 2018).

Thousands of demonstrators amassed in Los Angeles near Little Armenia to celebrate the 103rd anniversary of the Armenian genocide, which to this day Turkey maintains never happened. There were two marches, both of which were organized by the Unified Young Armenians. Participants waved flags and chanted to denounce the mass genocide of 1915 while calling for the US government to officially recognize it (Klemack, 2018). Instead of using the word "genocide," The White House has historically referred to the events that begin in Armenia in 1915 as "Meds Yeghern" (Great Calamity), which has been frustrating to Armenians (White House Statements and Releases, April 24, 2018).

As a hypothesis, it seems as though the projections onto the Armenians have not been "taken back." The Turkish people still deny that the genocide occurred. Hence, repair has not been possible because of massive denial. There is no possibility of healing that which has not occurred, so disparagement, hatred, and animosity prevail. Perhaps the change in leadership in Armenian will set the tone for change.

References

Address to a Joint Session of Congress and the American People (2001, September 20). United States Capitol, Washington, DC.
ADST. (2015, November 17). South Africa's Truth and Reconciliation Commission. *Huffington Post*, blog.
Al Jazeera. (2015, September). Rwanda: From hatred to reconciliation: The story of the 1994 Rwandan genocide told through the prism of the media, exploring their role then and today. Al Jazeera World.
Alford, C. F. (1989). *Melanie Klein and critical social theory: An account of politics, art, and reason based on her psychoanalytic theory*. Chelsea, MI: Bookcrafters, Inc.
Arlin, M. (2011). Honoring Odile Gakire Katese. In *Global Citizen*.
Casey, N. (2016, October 8). Colombia's President, Juan Manuel Santos, Is Awarded Nobel Peace Prize. *The New York Times*.
Dallaire, R. (2003). *Shake hands with the devil: The failure of humanity in Rwanda*. New York, NY: Carroll & Graf Publishers.
Freud, S. (1920). *Beyond the pleasure principle*. New York, NY: Norton Press.
Klein, M. (1946). Notes on some schizoid mechanisms. *International Journal of Psychoanalysis*, 27, 99–110.
Klemack, J. C. (2018, April 24). Flag-waving marchers in Los Angeles demand recognition of Armenian genocide. *NBC News*.

Merlino, G. (2014, December 9). Aleta Baun protects her Timor Indonesian homeland. Eden Keeper.

Sebaranzi, J. (2009). *God sleeps in Rwanda: A journey of transformation.* New York, NY: Simon & Schuster.

Seymour, L. J. (2007, October 11). Rwandans weave baskets of hope. *The New York Times.*

Sigri (2010, April 7). Rewarding Rwanda. Umuganda-Community Service.

Tumwebaze, P. (2015, October 23). Remarkable changes: Rwanda. *The New Times.*

White House Statements and Releases. (2018, April 24). Statement by the President on Armenian Remembrance Day. The White House. Retrieved from www.whitehouse.gov/briefings-statements/statement-president-armenian-remembrance-day-2018/.

Yerman, M. G. (2012, November 12). Sweet dreams: Reconciliation in Rwanda at DocNYC. *Huffington Post.*

PART V

Attempting to turn things around

From projective identification (a one-mind process) to mentalization (a two-minds process)

12

TREATMENT OUT OF THE ANALYTIC BOX

Attachment, mentalization, and a response to trauma

This chapter focuses on one of my major assertions that is shared by a growing number of philosophers, attachment theorists, psychoanalysts, and scholars, all of whom understand the importance of learning from experiences with others: people can only know themselves when they have been understood by another who has mirrored back to the subject his or her interpretation of the self. This suggests that people change not because of evidenced-based strategies alone that are used by therapists to help them recover from abuse, neglect, or other types of trauma. They change instead by "taking in" a new attachment figure. This new relationship forms a foundation of security and trust that can eventually lead to mentalization. If we accept that people design themselves after others, in the therapeutic setting it is the quality of the relationship that is most significant.

In the case of a diagnosis involving trauma, evidence-based research suggests that reliable results can come from working with exposure techniques, i.e. drawing patients mentally closer and closer to the experience of the traumatic event in the hope of desensitizing and eventually ridding them of the pain they endured. That's one approach; it works for some but is excruciating, even unbearable for others.

Another, more gentle way of working with people who have difficulties with exposure techniques is for a patient to have a present-moment experience with another, an intersubjective moment, one that strengthens the attachment to a therapist while making the connection more secure. Perhaps one way to achieve this goal with traumatized patients is by initially using metaphor and through storytelling, theirs and the others.

> The evolution of the human brain is inexplicably interwoven with the expansion of culture and the emergence of language. Thus, it is no coincidence that human beings are storytellers ... Thus, I believe that both the

urge to tell a story in our vulnerability and to be captivated by one are deeply woven into the structure of our brains … Emerging narratives begin to organize the nascent sense of self and become the bedrock of our sense of self in interpersonal and physical space … The role of language and narratives in neural integration, memory formation and self-identity makes them a powerful tool in the creation and maintenance of the self (Bruner, 1990). Stories are powerful organizing forces that serve to perpetuate both healthy and unhealthy forms of self-identity. There is evidence that positive self-narratives aid in emotional security while minimizing the need for elaborate psychological defences.

(Cozolino, 2010, pp. 163, 166–167)

In *Neuroscience of Psychotherapy: Healing the Social Brain*, Cozolino (2010) also highlights the importance of the co-creation of stories that can progress in complexity over time; new stories can be added to one's collection and older stories can be edited. Through the process of writing, modifying, and reorganizing narratives with patients, he believes that changes in life can occur (I do as well).

Instead of relying solely on cognitive strategies such as exposure techniques to draw patients mentally closer and closer to experiences endured during a traumatic event in the hope of desensitizing them, perhaps providing a safe, attachment-inducing base through the use of narrative might be more optimal—telling a story about "righting" a capsized boat and bringing a passenger safely back to shore might be more likely to lay the groundwork on which a solid alliance and secure base can be built.

As the relationship develops, one might help a person who has been traumatized develop images of, say, going near the water and then out on the water with a friend on a beautiful day, a day with a slight breeze at dusk, to share a magnificent sunset. One additional question is useful to explore: can a person who has been traumatized recover without developing (or rediscovering) the capacity to mentalize? Werner Bohleber (2010), among others who have been in the research trenches studying the early development of the self, says no. Instead he thinks:

> Modern research [indicates that] one's early mentalizing processes postulate a self that can only materialize by being mirrored by the psyche of the primary object: we need another person in order to experience our own self. Such a conception of self-emergence has its parallels in philosophical and sociological thought, by which it has, indeed, been influenced. Here we arrive at a level of reflection—the societal, cultural, intellectual, and philosophical currents of a given period—to which the changes in analytic theory and technique can be related.

(Bohleber, 2010, p. xvii)

If this is how the self is created, is a similar process necessary, in the case of a traumatized person, to re-establish one's selfhood? What types of experiences will make someone feel whole again—or more whole for the first time? With regard to the concept of trauma, there is a difference between trauma in general and PTS (post-traumatic syndrome), because technically speaking, the latter only involves military veterans. When it comes to treatment, it seems to me that most techniques used today have been selected from the same cognitive basket.

I, on the other hand, have treated traumatized people with success for many years doing something else. I could have and often planned to refer these patients to a trauma specialist; I had consultants lined up with phone numbers right by my side in case I ever needed them, and I did seek consultations now and again. However, much to my amazement, I rarely needed to make any such calls. And my patients got better. Why and how did that happen? I scratched my head for a few years as I wondered about this phenomenon, not knowing exactly why people improved. With so much specialization in the treatment of trauma, how was my ordinary daily practice succeeding?

Then, out of the unconscious blue, I began to think that it was the "end game" that really mattered: what a successful treatment looked like at the end of the day was the important part. I realized that I was approaching the dilemma of selecting treatment options from another direction: bottom-up versus top-down. I believe I listed mentally what I thought a traumatized person would need to live successfully after termination and went from there. I knew attachment was important. I thought some teaching would be necessary as well; teaching my patients how to calm down during extremely anxious times, as well as showing them other simple coping skills, all of which became an important part of my work. Through the combination of learning to know themselves while being able to trust another person as they acquired the ability to better regulate affect, my patients discovered (or rediscovered) their sense of self in a fuller sense of the word.

I also used an idea borrowed from Melanie Klein's (1946) description of babies' initial separation from their mothers, when they started to exhibit behaviors that indicated they had their own minds. I found that I practiced "my mind versus the mind of the other" within my own family. When my brazen 12-year-old daughter would say curtly, "Mom, *you* think it's stupid, but everyone who's cool thinks it's the best and I agree," or,

> Mom, I love you and you are pretty cool for a mother, but you can say dumb stuff, just stupid things. Why do I have to come home at one o'clock on prom night when everyone is staying out until after the sun rises? You're just old-fashioned. *You* want me to just stay home and not go at all.

At such moments I would stop what I was doing and ask a question. In this particular case that question would be, "whose mind thinks you should come home at one o'clock or not go at all, yours or mine? I don't think we've talked about this year's prom yet." I also found I was asking my husband similar "whose mind is it" questions, and much to my surprise he started to ask me the same thing. This question of "whose mind is it?" I came to refer to as the "one-mind process or a two-minds process."

Now I have these ideas in mind when I think about all of my patients' long-term needs, although my language is certainly different. This concept, I eventually realized, is not only a natural part of the way I work, it also incorporates mentalizing, what I have come to think of as applied mentalization. When I read Jon Allen's *Restoring Mentalizing in Attachment Relationships: Treating Trauma with Plain Old Therapy* (2013), I was greatly relieved because I was doing something similar. Allen's thinking about doing "plain old therapy" with patients who have experienced trauma seemed a lot like my way of working. One can use other techniques, but at the end of the day what makes people whole, what makes them healthy again? Allen's idea that people do best when they have a secure attachment and can learn to mentalize added to my sense that "treatment out of the analytic box" and "plain old therapy" helped people reacquire, or acquire for the first time, a sense of safety that allowed them to explore their inner as well as their outer environments, a process that set the stage for growth.

Even though I was not using the specialized evidence-based techniques that many therapists employ with traumatized patients, Allen's (2013) description validated some off-the-beaten-track approaches I've tried. For instance, I have strategies for "protecting" children from "the monsters under the bed" (for my own children it had been the anti-monster spray that worked best). Harry Potter has come in handy as well. One child was convinced that if she had Harry (one of my toy figures) with her when I was away, she would be protected because Harry's mother died so that he would be impervious to harm. With that "power" she thought he could protect himself and anyone with him, so she took the miniature Harry with her while I was away. One could say this strategy colluded with her magical thinking, that I gratified her wish instead of making an interpretation. However, the child did not wail for days as she had done previously. When I returned, we unpacked the events that had occurred during my absence. This patient came to understand that the Harry figure was a stand-in for me. She also came to know her feeling more fully and was able to eventually soothe herself versus needing me or Harry to do it.

With an adult patient I spent a couple of years imaginatively sailing on a pirate-proof ship with animals and no people. Eventually, when this quite traumatized but much improved patient was ready, we stopped by an island and started to pick up "people." Thereafter, real people entered this person's life one by one. This is the type of work I have done with very ill patients who have come to understand and process painful memories and associated conflicts that they eventually worked through. I have used other techniques as well when they have seemed appropriate, but always in the context of the larger treatment. Much like using one room for a specific purpose within a safe house, I have also created or cocreated individual stories with patients that eventually help them remember, talk about, and learn strategies for coping.

The emergence of redactional identification

What I am saying is that the new experience with a safe person allows for the development of something different. As a new state of mind emerges, it eventually becomes a conscious process that includes intention. A new element comes into play as the need for unconscious protection yields to awareness within the self-structure. This process one comes to know helps to solidify change. It is a conscious, known part of one's self that involves more than eradicating deplorable elements of one's being or tolerating one's own aggression. More than "getting rid of" or "putting up with" or "coming to endure" an unwanted part of the self, this new intentional process involves awareness of creating a new version of an old story. I am calling this newly developed, conscious process *redactional identification*, i.e., a way of creating a desirable aspect of one's self, learned at least in part from another person, perhaps directed by Alford's (2016) benevolent "inner other." This "inner other" is an active, knowable, and creative part of one's inner being. This concept appears to be related to Cozolino's (2010) idea about the importance of narratives and how new neural networks are formed: "Thus, I believe that both the urge to tell a story and our vulnerability to be captivated by one are deeply woven into the structures of our brains." He goes on to say:

> Therapy attempts to create this metacognitive vantage point from which shifting states of mind that emerge during day-to-day life can be thought about … You can begin by making clients aware of more than one narrative arc of their life's story and then help them understand that change is possible and offer alternative story lines. As the editing process proceeds, new narrative arcs emerge, as do possibilities to experiment with new ways of thinking, feeling and acting. The importance of unconscious processes of both parents and therapist is highlighted by their active participation of the co-construction of new narratives of their children and parents … In essence, therapists hope to teach their clients that they are more than the present story but can also be editors and authors of new stories.
>
> *(Cozolino, 2010, p. 171)*

References

Alford, C. F. (2016). *Trauma, culture, and PTSD*. New York, NY: Palgrave Macmillan.
Allen, J. G. (2012). *Restoring mentalizing in attachment relationships: Treating trauma with plain old therapy*. Washington, DC: American Psychiatric Association Publishing.
Allen, J. G. (2013). *Mentalizing in the development and treatment of attachment trauma*. London: Karnac Books.

Bohleber, W. (2010). *Destructiveness, intersubjectivity, and trauma: The identity crisis of modern psychoanalysis*. London: Karnac Books.
Bruner, J. S. (1990). *Acts of meaning* (Vol. 3). Cambridge, MA: Harvard University Press.
Cozolino, L. (2010). *The neuroscience of psychotherapy: Building and rebuilding the human brain*. New York, NY: W. W. Norton & Company.
Klein, M. (1946). Notes on some schizoid mechanisms. *International Journal of Psycho-Analysis, 27*, 99–110.

13

THE LADY—AS MY OBSERVING EGO—AND I

Observing mentalization after forming attachment relationships

When an uncle of mine moved to the West Coast, I inherited a few things from his law office, one of which was a tapestry. I learned later it was a replica of one of *The Lady and the Unicorn* tapestries, the originals of which are located in the Cluny Museum in Paris. The tapestry's true significance has been lost over time, but there are hints about its various meanings that are peppered throughout history. Many historians are in general agreement that the first five tapestries depict in some way the meaning of life (Davenport, 2011), a fitting role for the one in my office.

Although it was beyond my conscious awareness prior to my investigation of its meaning, perhaps the allegory depicted in "The Lady" was a harbinger of my good fortune, i.e., to have the opportunity to help people, young and old, search for and then find their own freedom. As I read more about the specific meaning of the unicorn tapestries, I learned that scholars believe their designers, as represented by the characters depicted within them, grappled with "Franchise," which represented the virtue of *liberum arbitrium* (Davenport, 2011). Loosely defined, this virtue was in some way related to self-awareness and moral freedom, helping one decide whether to choose desires associated with the natural appetites of the lion or pure reason associated with the unicorn (Davenport, 2011).

In the world of psychoanalytic thinking, one might conceivably compare Freud's ideas about the id and the ego to the lion and the unicorn. In Freudian parlance the struggle is between the desires and basic urges of the id and the reasoning functions of the ego, components of the personality that see to it that socially acceptable id demands are met in realistic and appropriate ways. Defense mechanisms of the ego help protect a person from socially undesirable id demands. At times, employing defense mechanisms of the ego to rein in or take flight from id impulses could be thought of as parallel to the struggles between the lion and the unicorn.

That being said, over the years, the "Lady" and I have assisted people in their search for meaning, I as a therapist, and the "Lady" as a metaphor from which others could learn how to weave together aspects of their lives. In many cases, the present-moment experiences "we" have had with patients have been the most rewarding, those times when something became known for the first time. It was then that something new was created.

Together we have had the privilege of watching the human psyche soar and have been there when some have plummeted to the depths of despair. In this space we have experienced every emotion men and women have known. It was as if we've been in storms in the West Indies and at times have glimpsed nirvana. Most cherished of all are the connections we've made and the help we've given to others who have walked down a similar road. You are a great inspiration, my Lady; you have become part of my soul.

The Lady and I have learned what human beings need to thrive and what holds them back in the grip of isolation. We've met terror as well as hope, powerful states that can lead to change throughout life. Inspired by the Lady I have learned how attachment, trauma, and mentalization are part of the same continuum. I also came to believe that a person needs to have certain capacities to be content with his or her life, capacities I consider essential if one is to thrive. This includes what Jon Allen (2013) has said on the topic, including the importance of having a relationship with one's self.

Because it is so crucially important to understand what children need to develop optimally (this applies to adult patients later in life if they were not exposed earlier to essential factors that make psychological environments safe), it is essential to know what it takes to create conditions wherein mentalizing can emerge (Allen, 2003). In this regard, it is fortunate that there is a fair amount of research that helps to inform us how mentalizing emerges (Allen, 2003; Allen & Fonagy, 2014). Infant observation helps us understand how this capacity develops as well.

Important ideas for parents and educators

First and foremost, children need to be loved, i.e., unconditionally loved, by parents. This does not mean parents need to agree with everything their children do, but rather that they need to accept a child's right to have an interpretation of his or her own without interfering. It is important for children to be able to have opinions without feeling they will be ridiculed or shamed (for patients, unconditional love is most appropriately replaced by unconditional respect).

I also believe that children need to know what it is like to trust, to be trusted, and to feel secure in a loving environment where certain behaviors are a part of everyday life. Key elements, acquired to a large extent through identification with primary caregivers, that are needed in an optimal environment for children (or adult patients) include empathy, honesty, compassion, patience, flexibility, integrity, and humility. It is also important for children to observe healthy ways of dealing with conflict and aggression. Self-awareness and self-reflection are important traits for them to come to know through observation, as is the capacity to be vulnerable, the capacity and freedom to be curious, and the capacity to be optimistic. Another characteristic that is essential for optimal development is the ability to mentalize. This is the capacity to know and respect one's own experiences as well as the experiences of others without judgment. One need not agree with another person's view of the world and can certainly engage in healthy debate, but the acceptance of the other's right to have a different opinion is important. In general, it appears that it is through experience and identification with others that this state of mind comes into being.

I believe, following John Bowlby's work, the most effective way to help a child develop the capacity to mentalize is by providing him or her with a secure attachment relationship from the beginning of life (Allen, 2003). When an infant can reach out to a primary caregiver for comfort in times of distress and consistently be soothed, he or she begins to feel secure. Regular and consistent contact with a loving caregiver creates an environment of security. Confident that an attachment figure can be depended on for help if needed, securely attached infants begin to be curious about their surroundings and explore their worlds on their own at very young ages, as has been observed by attachment researchers for decades. These researchers have watched young children as they venture away from their primary caregivers to explore all kinds of toys. When there is a secure attachment, they explore not only their outer worlds but also their inner worlds (Allen, 2003).

Returning to my work, 20-plus years into my practice, the Lady was my guide as I wrote a paper for a presentation in Barrie, Ontario. It was while preparing that document that I realized there could be positive possibilities in projective identification. That there was despair was obvious to me, but I also began to see how hope could be part of the process as well.

Some of the people we've met: Janie and Dr. J

The Lady and I spent many hours trying to assess and then help people of all ages come to know that they are individuals apart from anyone else. When all goes well, this work can be very rewarding. One case that comes to mind involved working with Janie. Janie and her mother, Dr. J, were very close. Each referred to the other as "my best friend." Two peas in a pod, they said. They dressed alike, sounded similar, and had the same haircut. Janie wanted to be just like Mom, and she got no resistance regarding her wish. Their relationship changed, they said, right after the accidental death of Janie's father and Dr. J's husband.

They were a team, that is until Janie was ten years old and arrived in my office one day with a brochure for a 12-week summer camp. On that day she was beside herself with excitement. She talked for the whole session about all the things she could learn at camp. When it was time for her to leave, her mother arrived. Janie raced to meet her to tell her about her plans, only to be met with tears.

"Why would you ever want to do that? It's hot and sticky and the girls aren't nice. I never did that," was Dr. J's initial response. Crestfallen, Janie slumped to the floor and cried so much she could hardly catch her breath. When they left, Janie looked distraught. That was the last session before the summer break. During the following year, after their vacation, which was spent in a cottage in Vermont, Janie seemed to be a different child. The bounce was out of her step. She did not seem like the girl who had been in my office the previous May.

We continued the treatment for two more years after she returned, but the tenor of our work together was quite different. She was no longer the curious child who wanted to explore the world. Instead she was serious and very apprehensive about her future. Rather than wanting to play imaginative games she had created, upon her return Janie wanted to do her homework. She was much more serious and she was very anxious.

Eventually I learned she had been very upset for most of the summer, but eventually improved after promising her mother that she would never go away to camp. During a session after the 1st of the year, Janie was extremely upset about an upcoming state-wide test she was scheduled to take in February. She described feeling as though she was being pressured about studying. When I tried to inquire about the source of the pressure, she became extremely anxious. She said, "Dr. M, not you too. I'm hard enough on myself and my mother is worse, but I usually get a break here." Not being certain what had triggered that response, I said, "Hm, it sounds like what I said bothered you." Janie replied, "You just sounded harsh and sarcastic and I don't expect that from you." Perplexed by her sense of my statement, I decided to wait and see what surfaced. In a minute or so she said, "I let you off the hook but you really are like her." I said, "Hm, tell me. Tell me your perception." To this Janie said, "You're being all high and mighty now. And you pressure me. You are just subtler, but you do it. We used to have fun here and I was learning things about myself. Now you're like a drill sergeant." I said, "Hm, tell me more about that," at which time Janie stomped away and went to the testing table. She said, "I know. I know I have to get this done."

After she was organized, with her things neatly placed on the table, I said, "So you feel I pressure you? Hm, I wonder." She said "Oh, stop it. You know you think that, even if you didn't say it. I'm lazy now. I get it." I waited. During the silence I realized that Janie was unaccustomed to anyone giving her space or letting her have her own thoughts without trying to replace them. Since her father died, I imagined. From what I gathered, their lives were good before the tragedy occurred. Unfortunately, Dr. J made sure they were both constantly busy after the death. They didn't have the opportunity to mourn the loss of their father and husband.

After Janie announced that she wanted to go to camp for the summer, Dr. J had trouble keeping things together. Finally faced with the death of her husband, she became very depressed. Janie felt guilty and vowed to do everything she could think of to make her mother better. This included not looking happy, not spending time with anyone except her mother, and making sure she only got A-pluses. After her comment about being lazy, I said, "So let me make sure I understand. You think I believe you should come here and do homework because you will fall behind if you don't because you are lazy?" She said, "More or less, you didn't say all that but you think it." I responded by saying, "Well let's think about this. We know who thinks that for sure without guessing or speculating. We don't know about the other person." "That's true," she said with a puzzled look on her face.

Toward the end of that session, I observed what seemed to be a turning point in the treatment. It was as if a lightbulb lit up the room as she began to question her thinking. She said, "You mean you *don't* think that? I thought if I thought it and my mother thought it, then you would think it, too. I don't really know why I thought that, you aren't really like her at all."

After the day Janie "got it," things shifted for her. She was clearer about what she needed and seemed to enjoy saying to her mother, "Who thinks that, you or me?" After it came together in her mind that she had her own mind that was different from her mother's or mine, she seemed to experience herself in a new way. She also became freer to state what she thought without being consumed with taking care of her mother or copying what she did or said—behavior that had emerged, at least in part, to assuage her guilt—initially over loving her father, which had not been a welcome or popular thing to say, and later because she had been "disloyal" by wanting to go to camp for the summer.

To summarize:

- The only man in this story is the father, to whom Janie had a deep attachment before it was abruptly cut off.
- Janie was seriously traumatized by his death; the chance to mourn was taken away from her, further interrupting her development.
- Dr. J, in lieu of mourning, projected her own self, with all its insecurities and demands for perfection, onto Janie, who fully identified with it.
- Blocked in developing her own sense of self, Janie eventually projected her mother's imposition onto me.
- After Janie recovered her stunted ability to mentalize, she was able to see herself as a separate person, to mourn, and eventually to understand her mother's difficulties without blaming her. She gained the self-awareness and the capacity to be self-reflective.

The couple

Then there was Monica and Charles. They came in ready to call it quits. Charles was raised in the South. His parents were heirs to a tobacco fortune. They were philanthropists and traveled around the world looking for causes they thought were worthy of their blessing. In their absence, several nannies raised Charles. His experience with them was positive. He said he had every need met when he was a child.

Since he was with them for most of his waking hours, the nannies had a major impact on his development. He reported that Ellie was the one in charge. She was tall, thin, and very opinionated. "What Ellie said was the way it was." When she had an opinion, it became a fact. Nobody challenged Ellie. Her word was the law of the land. At the same time, Ellie was "nice as pie," according to Charles. When he was sick, which seemed to be a frequent occurrence, Ellie served him in bed. He said he felt like a king. When his parents whizzed into town, they "fussed over him" and worshiped him as if he were a little prince. He rarely got into trouble because they protected him. He reported that he was a good kid, with one major focus: he aimed to seek adoration, to be thought of as the noble, gentle, and kind prince who would do anything for his people.

Charles's view of the world was fixed. He had many dos and don'ts that he would regularly recite. He could sound like a computer with a voice function, spouting facts, one after the other. One surprising observation was that he didn't sound as obnoxious as one might imagine. To my surprise, I really liked both of them. That's not particularly unusual for me, but most often liking patients was only part of the equation. I also had come to count on having access to my other feelings, i.e., sadness, hope, anger, joy, frustration, etc. With these two, however, there was something different. I only felt that I liked Charles and Monica as a couple. Usually, droning on and on about one's point of view is irritating to me; with this couple, it wasn't.

Monica was a mover. She knew what she wanted in life and was going after it. She was from a high-powered family in a city like New York City. She reported endless debates about business, politics, or anything else that had her family's interest and attention. This early exposure to different ideas led her to fight for her take on things. However, while she wanted her perception to be one of the items on the table, so to speak, she didn't seem insistent on her view exclusively. As we began working together, the tension mounted. Monica would get very angry when a conversation didn't include *her* sense of the situation or problem. The discussions would escalate quickly and then become very intense. And then, without my interventions, there would be long periods of silence.

After the work got underway, I noticed that I felt extremely tired, much more so than usual. Coffee did nothing to perk me up, nor did a walk prior to their session. Weeks turned into a month and the month felt like an eternity. I read all my saved articles from analytic training, from my own teaching, and from new books I bought. I just couldn't figure out why I liked them so much, yet found them so enervating.

And then one day it came to me. I wasn't observing two people sharing an opportunity to communicate with one another, I was watching a show. I felt like I was part of a performance but had no lines. When I "woke up," the music started to play. What I realized, with the Lady as witness, was their inability to mentalize; simply stated, each wouldn't or couldn't understand the views of the other. Although when I reflected on it, I recalled how effective Monica was at letting her thoughts be known. She differentiated her thinking from that of others, but somehow this capacity wasn't coming into the room in our sessions with Charles. She said the right things but something felt "off."

And Charles, that was a different story. He had gone on for months about what he thought about most everything. However, he didn't talk as if he were a know-it-all, as one might suspect; he just started to talk as if he were reading a grocery list. When this revelation finally came to me, I realized that, while I was sitting with two people who were "describing" aspects of their lives, I didn't have the sense that I was hearing people talk about their unique and individual experiences. When I made an inquiry about this, Charles looked at me as if he was hearing another language that he didn't understand. Monica, on the other hand, did know what I was alluding to. She said,

> He's like that, I'm used to it. I'm not sure he knows what you're talking about. His 'experience' reflects 'the facts.' I love him and that won't change, but there are things I have to do with my friends because he doesn't get that people have different views, not just his view.

As we continued to work I realized that Charles did not know that people come to this moment in time with their own set of experiences that are different from anyone else's; the subjective experience was not within his realm of understanding. He seemed to really believe that his experience of something was "the way things were." Clearly I had my work cut out for me.

We spent the next five years understanding what it means to mentalize; or, to revert to my former terminology that I introduce in Chapter 10, we learned about, "the one-mind and the two-minds process," i.e., a person knows about something in life because of what he or she has experienced up to this very moment in time. Another person has lifelong experience too, but it will never be our experience.

What I finally came to realize was that Charles didn't consciously know that other people have different experiences than his own that affect how they see and experience the world. Yet Charles did, for the most part, know Ellie's take on the world. He and Monica had never been able to get far enough in their discussions about much of anything because the communication between them would break down before they got to know how and why the other saw the world as they did. But Monica, being a mover, simply got involved in another project and busied herself with her friends, while Charles would give away money, something that made him feel good.

To compound the complexities in their relationship even more, Charles was a soft-spoken man who presented himself as a nice person. He was a wealthy man who was extremely generous. Beneath the generosity, however, Charles believed that he was right and other people were less informed because he knew the world as Ellie knew it.

To illustrate how sessions tended to go during the nearly six years that I saw them, I will include a session from our fifth year of therapy. Monica and Charles came in. They both looked frustrated. Monica said, "Ok, you tell him, I've tried and he doesn't get it. He won't ever get it because he can't, you can't make up for experiences someone doesn't have, he doesn't have any."

"I see how frustrated you are right now. What is it like for you not to feel understood?" I said. Monica replied, "Damn bad, that's how it feels. I don't think Charles can help it, though; he just spent too much time with the nanny and not enough with his mother. He doesn't know what he thinks." Charles joined in: "I get that she is frustrated, I am too. I know how you are supposed to live life, but I don't know how to comfort Monica when she needs something emotional."

"What's your sense of that?" I asked.

"Soothing. Ellie soothed me by rubbing my back or making me something to eat. I could do that, but I don't think that's what she wants and needs."

I said, "You learned a lot from Ellie, Charles. What comes to your mind when you think of how she made you feel safer or more loved when you needed to be comforted?" He responded by saying,

> She'd say she loved me and then would do something for me, like she'd take me to my castle fort and tell me a story about the prince who lived there or the knights who were brothers. If we were outside, we'd go to the castle with the moat. She would sing to me. She had a beautiful voice. She loved me. She was my real mother, not biologically speaking, but in terms of being attuned to me.

During this session, it was striking to me how much the nanny did for Charles when he was a young child. It felt as if she was taking care of a little prince while wearing kid gloves. So I said, "It seems as though Ellie did a number of things for you for which you've been forever grateful, but you couldn't be a little boy, you had to be a special child who never got dirty." To this Charles said, "I wanted to get dirty like the other kids and I wanted to play with them, but Ellie wouldn't let me. I was special and had to be put in a glass case." Charles then went on to describe how he always was given the "prince" role and he felt he had to do the same thing for women that Ellie did for him.

As it turned out, all of the jewelry Charles bought for Monica was an attempt to make her a princess as he had been made a prince. He wanted to show his love by adorning her with all of the princely things he had as a child due to his identification with Ellie and the way she loved and took care of him. This marked a turning point in the treatment. After the session, Charles began to understand that Monica wanted a partner and friend, not someone to idealize and praise her.

This shift led to more opportunities in the work to mentalize, to stand in the other's shoes while keeping a firm grip on how each felt about one thing or another. Each session was eye-opening as they both had new experiences with feeling loved, respected, and even cherished as opposed to feeling bowed down to or exalted. They became partners in the true sense of the word, accompanied by a subtle wink they created to signify that there were two minds in their group of two, not just one.

The Lady and I were relieved. We had witnessed the emergence of two well-functioning, separate people, each of whom had a greater capacity to love the other because they had the freedom to have and experience a self. They were two separate beings with an understanding of the self and the other.

To summarize:

- Charles had very little personal attachment to his parents, aside from inheriting their wealth and using it as they had (to borrow from Robert Frost): to procure "boughten friendship."
- He was attached to Ellie (although he cast her in a special role among multiple nannies orbiting around his princely self), but she seemed to have had little or no capacity to mentalize that would help him differentiate himself as a separate individual with his own mind.
- Ellie thoroughly projected her own puritanical standards onto him, and he identified with them so insistently that he could not imagine others' experiences and thus open himself up to well-grounded relationships.
- Monica's secure attachment to her family of origin provided her with a strong capacity to understand herself and others.
- Monica's capacity for mentalization was good, although she could hardly believe, at the outset of treatment, that Charles's was nearly nonexistent; she may have projected the success of her own early development onto him to some degree, and his resistance brought frustration for both.
- For both to stop playing roles that talked past each other was very difficult. It took effort for Charles even to realize what mentalizing meant once he began to change, while it was hard for Monica to realize that he could and would make changes. However, each eventually managed to see the other as a separate individual.

Camille's new voice

Grayson left Camille, making immediate plans for a divorce, because his father told him to "close that chapter in the book." Up to that point, Grayson had said that he loved Camille, that he was committed, and that he wanted to "be with her forever." But then her father-in-law, Dr. R, interfered, and on his say-so Grayson would no longer stay with her.

When the troubled communication between Grayson and his father began, the couple had tried to work together on their marriage. Dr. R's hostility meant they were dealing with a difficult situation as a loving couple. But they were empathic with each other, respectful of each other's needs, and aware that they needed to make time to be together rather than working all the time. (Camille had a good job as event manager and fundraiser for a Washington professional association.) They even discussed the prospect of having another baby, in addition to their four-year-old son, Josh. Camille thought—and felt—that her life up to that point had been ideal.

A week later, her world fell apart; she felt as if all joy was evaporating along with her husband. After Dr. R finally insisted that Grayson should leave his wife, there was no way to reach him. He was determined to go. "My father is right, and I never let myself admit it. This has been wrong from the start. He was right all along." With that Grayson left, found an apartment, and moved in; he gave up his job and went to work in one of his father's businesses. When he picked up Josh for weekend visits, he was filled with vitriol. Camille was stunned by the sudden, dramatic shift in his position.

Camille reported that the breath had been knocked out of her. She had been in love with Grayson since they were in college 15 years earlier and she still was. She had sensed that his parents, although pleasant to her face, didn't particularly like her, but the idea that they might dictate to Grayson to the point where he would leave her was not remotely on her radar. "Never in a hundred years did I imagine that my life would come to this." That she had been trying to get pregnant again seemed like a cruel joke—and very confusing. (Camille had wanted a girl; she said Grayson didn't care, and both couldn't have been happier at the prospect.) How could Grayson leave his son, his wife, and the possibility of a new baby? But leave he did.

As Camille told me when she began individual therapy several months later, the separation came about after she gave her parents money she had inherited from her grandparents in order to purchase a summer cottage as a retreat for the family. As the story unfolded, it became clear that Camille's maternal grandmother had left money for this dwelling in her will specifically as a legacy to Camille. They intended for Camille to keep and/or spend the money until she was established financially with her own family and income, no longer needing a nest egg. She had the right to spend these funds for college, her wedding, and/or for medical expenses until she reached her 35th birthday. Whatever was left was to go to her parents for the purchase of the cottage. Additionally, in her parents' will, Camille was to inherit the cottage when they were no longer able to live in it. The original funds themselves, plus monies for any tax and/or penalties, were left in the hands of a trustee who was to provide them to Camille when needed. In short, the matter was a legal contract within Camille's family, before she married Grayson.

When they initially discussed the upcoming transaction, Grayson seemed to agree it was something his wife needed to do; he appeared to be on board. During one early session Camille said with anguish that everyone knew the plan, and no one ever questioned it until Dr. R's opinion was made known. Only after Camille handed over the money to her parents did Grayson's father weigh in with full force; a week later Grayson, as it seemed to Camille, "changed his mind" and departed.

During the first three months after the separation she could not function. She had no interest in going out with friends, knew she was depressed, and looked for a therapist. That's when I initially met her. When she arrived in my office for the first time, it had been raining. When I went to greet her in the waiting room, she was wearing stylish rain boots, but otherwise was soaking wet. She was a bright, very attractive, 31-year-old woman who had a warmth about her that was very calming. When she sat down, the story about her recent experiences began to unfold. The immediate problem was finding a way to communicate with Grayson. Although she had thought they engaged easily until Grayson left, now she didn't know how to the process "the new Grayson." Camille found him often angry, sarcastic, and mean-spirited toward her. He refused to speak to her about virtually anything except picking up and dropping off Josh.

She said, "I don't recognize him. He's not the funny, smart, loving guy I knew; he's bitter. He rails at me for everything. I can't do or say anything that isn't immediately judged, then dismissed." Because of Grayson's new demeanor, Camille felt disoriented at times. She added,

> The other day when he brought over some tax papers, he asked me if I had made arrangements to sell the house. I thought I would pass out! We'd never discussed finances, division of property, or how Josh and I were to live. Who *was* this person? For four or five minutes, almost literally, I didn't think I knew him.

What was Dr. R's reasoning, a conviction powerful enough to cause this remarkable transformation in Grayson? Eventually he let everyone in both families know that it was his personal version of "community property": he thought that whatever Camille and Grayson brought into the marriage should belong to the couple, in both their names, which would preclude Camille disposing of "her" money as agreed. Apparently, it was "all about the money." But Dr. R added a nasty spin. He not only gave Grayson a hard time about Camille's fulfilling her grandparents' will, but said he would disown Grayson if he "let" his wife get away with this slick move. He also said,

> You can't trust blondes, especially blonde babes who are too big for their britches. You know, the ones who always butt into men's business. This decision is for the man to decide, and you are letting this woman drag you through the mud. Our family name is damaged. You better do the right thing.

Although I never met Dr. R, I found it easy to believe Camille's view that he resented her Ph.D. and her job. That he was a Lothario who had married for money seemed to be well known in their community. Grayson, who still referred to his father as "Daddy" when speaking to his mother, and who could not withstand the pressure of Dr. R's aggressive misogyny, adhered to his father's directive. He knew that "do the right thing" meant doing whatever it took to get rid of "pushy" Camille—or else. And he promptly (and, I guessed, somewhat guiltily) did so.

As the work with Camille got underway, I knew my initial impression was right: this was a competent, very smart person who was going through perhaps the toughest period she had experienced in her young life. As she spoke, I felt very empathic; I could only imagine what it must have been like for her. Although her depressed state kept her from expressing much affect, I sensed that she wanted help and knew she needed it. I guessed that people usually liked her, as I did. I also thought she was probably a good mother, which was reassuring: at least Josh would have a caring mother to help him through a rough time with a largely absent father.

After the initial shock of Dr. R's successful attack and Grayson's departure, Camille received lots of support from her friends, who took turns spending nights at her house because she was afraid to be alone. Her mother, Sally, rushed to town from a Western state to help her daughter as soon as she learned of the separation; she stayed for many months to take care of Josh, since the grief-stricken Camille barely got through each day. Worried about her son, Camille appeared to be experiencing some loss of her identity as a mother. Too depressed to engage much with Josh, she was scared that her low mood would affect him over the longer term. So she was very relieved that her mother could take over her childcare responsibilities for a while. While Sally was upset about Grayson's actions, according to Camille she also felt sorry for him. Her sympathy for him persisted even after, during a visit to the house, he starting throwing flowerpots at the walls.

Over the next year, the clinical picture became much clearer. Camille said she felt like half a person without Grayson. She mourned,

> He rounded me out: what I wasn't, he was. Now I'm like a wet cloth. I'm just kidding myself to think I can do it all without him. It's such a struggle to go through a day and then come home to nothing. He used to know what I was going to say before I opened my mouth. I think his strong personality influenced me; I didn't have to make decisions or stay on the fence about anything because he always knew the right thing to do. He was the conductor, and it sounds so stupid when I hear myself say these things, but it's what I think about all day—I can't do this without him.

I responded, "It sounds like you feel, in some ways, like you and Grayson are one person; you seem to feel incomplete without him. It's as if he's your oxygen; without him you can't survive." Quickly she said,

> But I'm an old women's-rights soul from way back. When I was a child I went with my mother on marches. Now I'm a disappointment to all women. Yes, that's what it feels like, and I hate being so dependent.

> I think my friends would like to say what you just did, but they don't want to hurt my feelings. I have to face this, though.

After that exchange, I let silence reign for a few minutes. Clearly Camille was having a pretty strong reaction to what I had said, and to the insight and realization in her answer. She needed time to process her experience; she cried profusely, then cried some more. When she did speak, she had reached a realization.

> Wow, I guess I'm saying I'm not alive without Grayson. I was a whole person just now, but with no one to rescue me. I guess I was waiting for you to bail me out of the abyss. But after a few seconds, I knew somehow you weren't going to do that, because you think I can do it myself. And you're right. Right then, a few minutes ago, I felt something almost physical, like an internal shift or something. Like I was growing, being stretched. Yes, I can do this. Because of Josh I still have to deal with Grayson, but I don't have to *be* him any longer.

After another period of pensive silence, Camille took a new tack, returning to an earlier self.

> When I was younger, people thought I was funny. I don't have to be a funny person now to match Grayson; I can find that funny kid in me that people laughed with when I did imitations. I think I was pretty good. I can be good again now, for me. This could almost be like a new beginning. I don't have to be Grayson, I can learn to really be Camille.

Following that session, Camille went to Sedona for a two-week work event that involved new people and ideas, with plenty of time for recreation. When she returned, she seemed excited about her life and ready to deal with the reality of her situation. This was the beginning of the search for the real Camille. Although she made jokes about "both Camilles," a new kind of awareness developed. She called her engagement and marriage the "me-him" period. Since Camille hadn't been compliant in earlier relationships in life, she decided there must have been something about Grayson that "sucked her in." She speculated that she had some need to help him shine, even at her own expense. As our hours passed, she reviewed items that popped into her head concerning where Grayson stood on things and where she stood, eventually deciding—sometimes with great astonishment—that the real Grayson and the real Camille were very different people.

Because it was so difficult for Camille to understand, then expel, Grayson's projection and reclaim her own persona, she stayed in treatment for another six years. We continued to work on the "kidnapping" of Camille: how it happened, how her internal world was affected by the takeover. She imagined what her life could be like when not with a man who knew everything, in a new place where she could soar. And she did soar, eventually becoming the executive director for a national association. Thereafter, Camille became the executive director of a major international human-rights group. Meanwhile, Josh grew into a cheerful, soccer-playing, trombone-playing teenager, the joy of his mother's life.

When I initially saw Camille, I hadn't yet read the word "mentalize" (nor, of course, had she). What we were focused on was a second person emerging from the shadow of the first person, one who had to gain the freedom to accept and embrace a mind of her own: a Camille made whole again. She thought she had had that freedom as an infant with her mother, her primary caregiver, and then with both her parents. She was thankful that both encouraged her to have her own thoughts and feelings; she realized what she had once had and almost lost: her own voice. Without blaming Grayson any more, and without judging him, she accepted that she had somehow allowed him to project himself onto her, then colonize her personality. Now she met men and enjoyed their company, but with a full life she did not remarry. When she left treatment, she was a whole person—as she put it, "a whole hot tomatillo," homegrown and delicious, rather than "a tasteless, hydroponically grown, unripe tomato from the grocery shelf."

To summarize:

- Grayson never hit Camille, but the violence he did to her life was as damaging as many blows.
- While I know nothing firsthand about Grayson's childhood attachment, the adult result makes clear that his father gave him "roots" but never "wings," and little capacity to grow and develop on his own. This is a classic case of projective identification with an engulfing father. Grayson could not mentalize or see Camille as a person separate from himself, and—projecting the phony-adult male he had absorbed from his father—he treated her viciously when she asserted her independence.
- Camille believed she had a good attachment in childhood, but she clearly retained some vulnerabilities that left her unprotected from Grayson's projections, i.e., projections of archaic ideas about a woman's role in society. Moreover, she fully identified with his image of her appropriate position (hence the persisting desire for a new baby), which leads to the most severe psychological damage.
- Given her strong identification with Dr. R's projection onto Grayson, Camille was traumatized by Grayson's sudden departure. She grieved as if it were a death in the family.
- Camille initially idealized Grayson but eventually was able to "give back the projections." This was a difficult task for her. In the end, she completed it well and began to live a happy, self-realized life.

A bright, smiling face and a train

The Lady and I once had the unique opportunity to meet a child who taught us a great deal. This person, J, was a five-year-old-boy. Sadly, he was HIV-positive when he came for his first session. During that first meeting and many times thereafter, he wanted to play with a small train set. There were toy people that went with this set, in addition to the train itself.

Each time he arrived and wanted to play with the train, he would go to the toy area to collect what he wanted to play with and would bring everything to the center of the room. He would then ask me to play with him. While he set everything up the way he wanted it to be, he would say a few times, "Don't panic, it will be OK. Don't panic." I would say things like, "Oh, I see. You want the people to feel better." He would respond by nodding his head to indicate that I was correct. At times he would again say, "Yeah, don't panic." Thereafter he would say, "Panic if you want to." He then would take the train, go down the tracks and hit the people. This all took place while he was laughing. When I'd ask him what happened, he initially would shrug his shoulders and say, "They panicked."

Eventually he expanded on what had gone wrong. He said that the people didn't listen so they got smashed. As we continued to work, it became clear that J was very angry and scared about his illness. Prior to being adopted by the couple who brought him to therapy, J heard lots of things that were said by his mother and her boyfriend. As I came to know more about his early years, I learned that he overheard his mother, who had been addicted to heroin, say things like, "He's going to die, just get used to it" or "It's OK, he's going to die." What became clear was that he experienced emotional pain and protected himself by putting it someplace else, e.g., he projected his angry feelings that were unbearable to him onto the train conductor. As long as he could hit people on the track, he could express his rage at made-up people who couldn't harm him.

As the therapy progressed, J was able to use words he knew to describe the feelings he had. This was more satisfying to him. It helped him have a better understanding of his feelings, helped him modulate his affect more effectively while feelings intensified between the two of us. The Lady and I tried to help others become who they wanted to be; not what we, another, or others wanted for them but what they wanted for themselves. This included J.

J died a year and a half later. At the end of his life he was much more able to express his feelings. He was able to use words to express himself. He was angry and sad and he was happy, too. In a remarkable way, he seemed to have some awareness that he wouldn't be here when he died but seemed to be comforted by the idea that people would remember him. Working with this child was a true gift.

To summarize:

- J's HIV (and perhaps addiction) at birth gave him the most physically damaged start to life a child can have.
- Living for a number of months with an addictive mother and her violent-sounding boyfriend provided him no emotional attachment whatsoever, but rather rejection.

- With no caregivers to model emotion and a sense of self, J turned to mechanical objects, projecting his overwhelming fear and anger onto them.
- Gradually, as he grew comfortable in his adopted family and was in treatment, he could retract those projections and begin to play with a doll family, to whom he ascribed emotions other than sheer panic.
- When he began to be able to speak of his own feelings, J developed a sense of himself, in relation to loving others, that made his last months brighter and less fearful.

References

Allen, J. G. (2003). Clinical implications of attachment and mentalization: Efforts to preserve the mind in contemporary treatment mentalizing. *Bulletin of the Menninger Clinic*, 67 (I), 91–112.

Allen, J. (2013). *Mentalizing in the development and treatment of attachment trauma.* London: Karnac.

Allen, J. G. & Fonagy, P. (2014). *The American Psychiatric Publishing textbook of psychiatry* (6th ed.). R. Hales, S. Yudofsky & L. Roberts (Eds.) Arlington, VA: American Psychiatric Publishing.

Davenport, A. (2011). Is there a sixth sense in the *Lady and the Unicorn* tapestries? *The New Arcadia Review, 4*, 1–15.

CONCLUSION

One recent morning as I pulled out of Savannah, with moss-dripping live oaks behind me and sea oats and marsh grass bringing the scent of the sea from my left, I thought about my personal "travels" and how I had gotten to my own "ports of call" in life. I was heading for the Overseas Highway again, going back to my home in the Keys with its palm trees, marlins, and pelicans. With a day's journey ahead of me, I began to think about my early professional life: how I'd gone from casually hearing about the Washington School of Psychiatry and its rich history some 35 years earlier to having had the good fortune to serve as the director of an important part of the School, the Meyer Treatment Center. I remembered an important call I received at the School from Bob Ursano, then the editor of the journal *Psychiatry*. I had met Bob some years before, when I was a candidate at a local psychoanalytic institute. I recalled thinking he was one of the best and brightest analysts there, as well as an impressive teacher.

The purpose of the call was to ask if I was interested in writing a commentary for a journal on one of Clara Thompson's articles from 1945, "Transference as a therapeutic instrument." Since the topic was central to psychoanalytic practice, and since Bob wanted me to write the piece, I immediately agreed. But while I was delighted to be asked, I soon realized that I knew little about Clara Thompson. Still, I knew I could write the article, so I set out to learn as much as I could about her. As I breezed through the tangle of highways in Atlanta, I recalled my puzzlement at learning that I was not the only person who was uninformed. I was dismayed to learn that Thompson had been all but forgotten, despite her important early contributions to psychoanalysis. As Paul Roazen said in his introduction to a new edition of Thompson's 1950 book (Thompson, 2003) *Psychoanalysis: Evolution and Development with a New Introduction by Paul Roazen*, "… the work of Clara Thompson remains in a kind of limbo, a no-man's land reserved for people who have seemingly vanished historically" (p. xiv).

Soon I grasped that Thompson was ahead of her time: while trying to preserve and expand upon many of the basic principles of classical psychodynamic thinking, she introduced new ideas—including those of Sándor Ferenczi—that are highly significant in today's relationalist climate. Thompson also took significant risks to go against the tide of traditional thinking. According to Aron (2001), she encouraged patients to talk about what they observed in their analyst, suggesting that such observations could lead to further insights on the part of the analyst, a current idea. Yet it is unlikely that analysts today would attribute contemporary thinking on countertransference or mentalization to Clara Thompson.

Gazing once again out of my car window toward Georgia's sea islands, I remembered how—once my commentary had been published—I initially began to write this book to bring Clara Thompson and her original ideas back to life. After reading as much as I could find about her contributions, I agreed with Roazen (Thompson, 2003), who charged historians with the task of reintroducing Clara Thompson and the neo-Freudians who bravely introduced ideas that went against the strict Freudian status quo, once-unwelcome ideas that have become commonplace. Thompson and her colleagues sacrificed to promote new observations about best therapeutic practice, requiring new psychoanalytic theory.

In the process of resurrecting my new heroine's contributions, I came across interesting letters she had written in her favorite South Sea blue ink. They were reminders of the everyday work she did, the "grit of the day" that spread her thinking among her colleagues during her lifetime. Contemplating Thompson's journey up close led me to a broader search, looking for the lives of other women who carried a banner for truth and justice but who also had not been adequately recognized or remembered. One such woman was Eleanor Marx, daughter of Karl Marx, who had championed the plight of women a century earlier, asking from a socialist perspective "what is to be done?"

As I sailed into Florida on I-95 with my destination on the far horizon, I remembered how I drew together the hypothesis that would give structure and meaning to my book: these gallant women whom I was coming to know suffered in very different ways from a common dynamic forced on them by others, frequently by a man or, more often, men. As a psychoanalyst and therapist, I had a lifetime of experiences that, considered systematically, suggested how those women—and sometimes those who have victimized them—might be helped. The problem, as readers now know, is projective identification, the unconscious thrusting onto another person of bad feelings that the subject cannot tolerate, which may or may not be perceived by the recipient of those emotions. If the recipient "accepts" and identifies with them, the projector may dream of creating a symbiotic state in which he or she can control the recipient. The resulting "relationship," based on fantasy, is painful for both participants.

A solution for some (if only their therapists knew about its power) is mentalization. I hope my examples have shown how personal, healthy relationships with others can develop. That process can begin when a strong therapeutic alliance is built and maintained between a patient and his or her analyst, leading to a secure attachment. In this way, people can recover or establish a capacity for mentalizing, which in turn can protect them from the fallout of projected and unwanted emotions or thoughts they received. Moreover, individuals who have identified with the damaging images thrust upon them—who have been "gaslighted" about their own personalities and contributions—can regain an accurate sense of self and maybe discover their "inner other" for the first time. In these individual cases, the goal of therapy focuses primarily on building or rebuilding a capacity for trust in order to heal damaged relationships or to build healthy, rewarding new ones. Treatment might have saved Eleanor Marx's life. Clara Thompson had more than one analysis; we can hope her experiences helped her gain some understanding of roadblocks that curtailed her distinguished career. Hillary Clinton, a very private person, seems to the public eye to have recovered her equanimity after her loss of the presidency; perhaps others have helped her relocate her "inner other" once again. No matter what the case may be, most people will never know how deeply she was wounded.

When entire groups of women or any other group of people have been subjected to projective identification, the challenge may be greater, in numbers alone and often in severity of violence. It takes enormous courage for victims like the "radium girls" to band together, find leaders and lawyers to give voice to the harm done to them, and seek recompense that can never be adequate. The oppressors who denigrated and denied them were corporate officers, corrupt physicians and dentists, and lazy bureaucrats. Many of these men could not imagine working-class women as their equals; most felt far more obligation to profits, growth, and (in today's language) shareholder value. Fortunately, progressive journalists and public-health scholars, often women, led the way in bringing the radium girls' plight to attention and, long after the fact, in establishing state and federal laws and agencies like the National Labor Relations Board (NLRB), the Consumer Products Safety Commission (CPS), the Food and Drug Administration (FDA), the Occupational Safety and Health Administration (OSHA), and the Environmental Protection Agency (EPA), which supervises chemicals released into air and water. But these agencies are not popular with employers and producers. Companies do not readily agree to inspection, testing, and prohibitions; they pay lobbyists vast sums to fight relentlessly (and under President Trump, successfully) against regulation. Serious harm in the workplace remains an ever-present danger (Greshko, Parker, Howard & Stone, 2018).

Passing the exit for Patrick Air Force Base, gleaming in the sun, I recalled the military men who projected disdain onto the WASP even while the women were in the air serving their country at war. Then congressmen exiled them from the air as the war was ending. The gender-stereotyping culture promptly hung out a NO WOMEN WANTED sign for all jobs in flying except, of course, that of stewardess. And the government refused to classify the WASP as a military service, apparently trying to eradicate from all memory the inconspicuous but heroic work they had performed. Decades later, refusal to inter the ashes of the WASP in military cemeteries (which would have acknowledged their service, by name) simply added to the insult. Although President Obama awarded these intrepid women a medal, the issue remains unresolved. It is way too late for therapy to help any of these women understand what caused her pain. Like the industrial damage to the radium girls, military assaults on the dignity of hardworking women can be alleviated by legislation and federal action. Eternal vigilance is the price. Fortunately, since Tailhook feminist campaigns have made some differences in the treatment of women by the military. Progress toward equality, however, is far from complete. The question remains: how thorough was the change in procedures (Ricks, 2017)?

As I continued my sojourn south, with shadows growing long on the ocean, I became keenly aware of the awesome juxtaposition between my childhood memories set in the tranquil Keys and the children of despair: those who had been exposed to the atrocities associated with human trafficking. In the case of sex-trafficked girls and women, the expertise and the networks of law enforcement—local, nationwide, and international—are obviously essential for rescuing the victims and for prosecuting and punishing the traffickers. But what can be done when police blame, even arrest, victims under 18 for prostitution? What happens when the public social services available to assist rescued girls with housing, food, medical care, and counseling are scant, short-term, or so inadequate that the girls feel compelled to return to the streets or brothels to support themselves—or their children, or their habits? What happens when projective identification is everywhere and hard to sort out?

Obviously, sustained intensive treatment should be available to help the girls recover a sense of self and gain some perspective on pimps. For this problem, urban civic services—perhaps especially Child Protective Services under various names—are necessary, but saddening news reports from many cities show that they are often understaffed by poorly qualified and overworked people with low morale (Sher, 2013). Many other problems compete with children's services for city funding, and states are not very likely to help. Private not-for-profits managed by people who understand the situations of girls at risk do excellent work, but they are a drop in the ocean of need. What happens when the media's brief attention span and the public's momentary titillation mean that sex-trafficking disappears from the headlines … until the next time? More civic-minded women who run for local office and persist in keeping this issue on the agenda might make a major difference.

Interethnic conflict in a small, shared space like Rwanda, especially when it leads to mass rape and genocide, is more difficult still to address. United Nations rules, commissions on human rights, and even convictions in courts on war crimes in the former Yugoslavia and West Africa have failed to deter vicious hatreds and their projection: see the degradation of Yazidi women and girls by ISIS in Iraq, or sexual enslavement by Boko Haram of girls (Searcey & Akinwotu, 2018) who have sought education in northeast Nigeria, or the rape and "ethnic cleansing" of Rohingya women in Myanmar (Nianias, 2018). Beyond the rise of reparative leaders on the victors' side, a spirit of truthful, nonpunitive reconciliation, and the empowerment of women—all of which seem immensely idealistic in the present climate—I have no solutions. But there is understanding. And that helps. It is a first step in a myriad of confusion.

As I drove to my destination, I realized why I felt compelled to go to Marathon, my former home and a Key located along Overseas Highway between Miami and Key West, before I finished my manuscript. There was something else I needed and I was certain I could find it there. Although I didn't know why at the time, I was right. One night during my visit, under a star-filled sky, it became clear to me that being on the receiving end of projective identification was similar to my experiences of being, "on the other side of the eye."

Being ripped, torn, and tossed around in a state of confusion is similar to "the other side of the eye" of a hurricane. As the projector rids himself of unwanted hatred, terror, and fear, the other is racked with confusion and uncertainty while being stripped of a recognizable self, due to a fantasy thrust upon him or her by another. This is like being in the second phase of a hurricane, after the eye passes. In both situations the force destroys the foundation (of one's inner being) and uproots everything in its path. Nothing is familiar, the words "what happened?" apply in both cases. In a devastating storm when everything is lost it is like being the recipient of a projective identification: the receiving person loses his or her bearings. In both circumstances, even if ever so briefly, one has nothing left, one is disoriented in that space because what is familiar is gone. The center of the self, the foundation of one's familiar being is no more, whether that person loses his or her external surroundings or internal being. In a hurricane one is frightened. Will it blow me away? Will I die? Will I be found? When in a projective identification one is faced with a cloud of confusion. Was that my thought or yours? Where did it come from? I don't know that idea, is it mine? It's crazy and unclear. I feel like I am in a fog. When all is said, and done, being in a hurricane is like being slammed with someone else's thoughts.

When one is in a hurricane, it can be very scary. The wind howls, objects are often lifted by the wind and moved from one place to another. Trees often break in half as water rises. There can be much destruction over a period of many hours. And then there is a period of calm. If one doesn't know how hurricanes progress, he or she might think it is safe again, that the danger has passed as when a thunderstorm is over. A person could be tempted to go outside to begin to assess the damage or start to clean up objects that have been tossed about. However, the storm is not over. The worst part is yet to come.

With these thoughts in mind, I looked up hurricanes that hit Miami and the Keys on my computer. I found just what I was looking for to illustrate an external event that appears to be akin to an internal phenomenon. It was told by Don Van Natta Jr. of the *Miami Herald* who was staying in a Comfort Inn in Florida City, Florida on August 24, 1992. He and his journalist colleagues, and other guests, having congregated, considered toasting to their first shared hurricane. After all, it hadn't been so bad, they thought. It was calm.

What they didn't know was that they were in the eye of the storm and for a while all was still. They opened their door and noticed silence. There was an eerie silence that permeated the space. This brief respite was followed by a series of sounds and pyrotechnics. "The other side of the eye" was there. Transformers began to explode, sending sprays of blue and green light across the night sky. Abruptly, the power failed. An hour went by, punctuated by sound effects included the shattering of glass and the screech of metal roofing peeling free; part of the motel's roof was ripped away. As the wind moaned ominously, the group made a beeline for another room, armed with flashlights and candles, but then water began to drip from the ceiling and they fled to yet another room.

Five a.m. arrived, and the drop in barometric pressure made everyone's ears pop; the sound of metal being mangled, hurled against things, grew more intense. Although the night was pitch black, cars in the parking lot were visible, and they had been dented, damaged, windshields were smashed. Then the hotel manager, a former Navy man, knowing that the wind would change direction, advised everyone to shift to the building's north side; this move probably saved their lives. The wind was surging at 165 mph, palpably violent, and the group dashed from room to room in search of safety. In one of the rooms cracks appeared in the ceiling and plaster began to come loose; it seemed near collapse. But they were trapped: the wind's pressure had sealed the door shut. Nine people squeezed into the bathroom; they heard an explosion and water began to trickle in. People panicked, pressed together, prayed aloud, and did their best to shore up the buckling ceiling. Plaster fell to a deafening rumble outside. Finally, the pressure eased, the door could be opened, and the group dashed to room 240, where they encountered the manager and a few of the motel's other occupants.

As it began to get light, the group peered outside and saw that most of the motel had been blown away. Van Natta left the premises and began to explore what remained of Florida City. Rain-soaked residents staggered out of badly damaged houses. Ninety percent of the town was destroyed; with no landmarks to guide them, people were disoriented in their own neighborhoods. The town awaited the hurricane's aftermath, which would include the arrival of the National Guard and insurance-company assessors, the erecting of tents. Van Natta and his fellow reporters piled into the photographer's battered car, which, miraculously, started, holding towels in front of their faces as protection against flying shards of windshield glass. They drove north through a ravaged landscape and filed their story at the headquarters of the *Miami Herald*. Van Natta has kept his room key as a souvenir.

Projective identification, as the other example of losing one's bearings, is also dangerous. It is a tricky maneuver primarily because the early phase of the process starts out with a fantasy of one person that is foisted onto another: it is someone else's idea about us. It is not what we think of ourselves but rather what someone else believes about us and is really about the person who is doing the projecting.

This dynamic is further illuminated in the following example; one I recalled after reading about the 1992 hurricane. "He yanked my purse out of my hand, opened it and threw everything on the floor while calling me a 'A stupid, greedy bitch'." Jessica was numb, she didn't know what was happening. She was afraid to breathe. Jason went on ranting and raving, saying she'd robbed him of everything he'd ever had in life. More perplexed than ever, Jessica sat down on a pillow he'd thrown on the floor. Her body was shaking. The rant continued as her sense of safety on the floor vanished. She tried to figure out what had led to this outburst as she sat trying to pretend she was a silent, still statue. Fear of disturbing Jason as he continued to depict her as a despicable character seemed to get a grip on her. She began to wonder whether or not she was a dishonest, bad person for upsetting him. Had she stayed out too late, did she talk to his friends too much? Did she think of herself too much, as Jason claimed?

The first phase of this process consisted of a fantasy that the projector had to shed. He had to get rid of a "bad" part of himself that he could not tolerate. However, the ridding of that unwanted part was only partial. There was also a wish to keep tabs on what was projected in an attempt to control the other person. In this way, the projector creates and maintains a symbiotic-type fusion with the other, allowing him or her to maintain a sense of oneness with the recipient. Once this is achieved, the projector unconsciously tries to pressure the recipient into behaving in a way that fits his or her fantasy. If the recipient responds, a two-body process of projective identification occurs. The recipient is expected to behave in a way that is congruent with the projector's fantasy.

Having discovered more about myself, hurricanes, patients I have met, and projective identification, I headed back to the mainland. As I took in the beauty of my childhood haunts, I remembered my first journey to my current home. It was one filled with excitement about a new world; a place where I could really grow up. It was there that I found my own true voice with the help of so many. I was exposed to a sea of knowledge and experiences that helped me learn how to help others find their own voices. It was there that I learned more fully about the concept of mentalization, which is an essential part of the process of growth and change. It was in my new, grown-up home that I learned that people can revise earlier versions of themselves.

This way of revising oneself, which I have called "redactional identification," evolves through a process of editing old ways of being, leading to the creation of new aspects of the self. As one learns to navigate differently in the world with the help of another person, usually a therapist, he or she comes to know and appreciate the value of actively participating in life with *intention*.

It is similar to Cozolino's (2010) idea of therapy, i.e., by helping clients realize that their current life is not the only possible way in which to live, one can embolden them to create other narrative arcs. They learn that they can be the authors of different stories about their own lives (Cozolino, 2010). Living life with intention highlights the importance of learning from others, which is closely linked to attachment theory. It also incorporates Prinz's ideas about agency and intentionality, features which he suggests arise from interactions with others (Prinz, 2012).

I returned my rental car, boarded the airplane, and headed north filled with excitement once again about the internal adventures I had in the Keys and a renewed readiness to continue learning while helping people come to know the destructive power of projective identification as well as the possibilities that can emerge from secure attachments and mentalization.

As the airplane was taking off, the pilot made a shallow climbing bank to the right on the way to a cruising altitude of 30,000 feet. After passing through a line of clouds, the airplane emerged into clear skies. From my seat near the window I could see an outline of part of the Keys. How fortunate I was, I thought to myself as I pondered my old world filled with childhood adventures that were accompanied by a sense of freedom to wonder. I knew then that my varied and rich opportunities in the Keys set the stage for the understanding I now have of the self I know and of others that I have encountered in my life as a woman, a psychologist, and a psychoanalyst.

In that regard, I believe we are the sum total of what we have experienced up to this very moment in time. As individuals making our way in a world filled with unimaginable beauty on one end of the continuum and incomprehensible pain on the other, as well as everything in between, we can only know what we have experienced, and what we have come to know from others, nothing more. The subjective experience reigns supreme.

Firmly ensconced once again in my Washington, DC, world, I thought about recent gains as well as disappointments while entertaining prospects of hope. Gains include one of this year's Nobel Peace Prize winners and the reason she won. Nadia Yousafzai, a former sex slave held by ISIS, was recognized for her efforts in fighting sexual violence; acknowledging her heroism was a major step forward for the Nobel Prize Committee. In physics, Donna Strickland, only the third woman to win this prize in 117 years, shared her award with Gérard Mourou for their work in laser physics (Brumfiel, 2018). After hearing about this year's winners, I had to wonder if earlier projections of prejudice had been "taken back," allowing for repair and the emergence of a more judicious and fair-minded process.

Problems, however, continue to exist within the Nobel Committee. Internal scandals about sex-abuse allegations roiled and divided the ranks, who didn't award a prize in literature this year; seven of them, in fact, quit—despite having lifetime appointments (Heintz & Lewis, 2018).

Then there is the travesty that occurred with the appointment of Brett Kavanaugh to the Supreme Court. In spite of the heart-wrenching testimony of Dr. Christine Blasey Ford, whom many senators believed regardless of party affiliation, Kavanaugh became a Supreme Court Justice before a thorough investigation of the allegations made against him could be conducted. Perhaps the most appalling moment in this ordeal came when President Trump openly mocked Dr. Blasey Ford, who told her painful story of sexual assault before the Senate as well as millions of people around the world who saw the broadcast.

It would appear that Donald Trump once again resorted to projective identification as he spewed his verbal venom onto Dr. Blasey Ford and the public in order to distance himself from his earlier statements that indicated he thought she was a fine woman who was very credible. While the President's positive remarks resembled the early steps of mentalization, in which one appears to accept and respect what is on another's mind, this brief shift in his usual negative stance turned out to be disappointing to many people who believe truthfulness matters. As a hypothesis, it seems as though President Trump had to get rid of good thoughts about Professor Blasey Ford because he could not tolerate having conflicting or ambivalent notions about her. Instead of having positive as well as negative ideas about this woman, holding both impressions in his mind, he had to disavow his emerging sense of her honest testimony by disparaging her. In this way he regained praise and admiration from Republican Senators as well as his base—those Americans who support him regardless of the content of what he says—as exemplified by the cheers he received from a crowd at the rally where he made fun of Dr. Blasey Ford.

We do not know if Donald Trump will ever be able to turn a corner, so to speak, and "take back" the many and varied projections he has forced onto others or whether he will eventually take responsibility for his actions. If he were able to learn how to seriously consider and respect the thoughts and ideas of those who have different opinions, a move toward hope, repair, and reconciliation could be possible wherein misogyny and projective identification could give way to mentalization.

References

Aron, L. (2001). *A meeting of minds: Mutuality in psychoanalysis.* Mahwah, NJ: Lawrence Erlbaum Associates, Inc.

Brumfiel, G. (2018, October 2). The Nobel Prize in Physics: 117 years, 3 women and counting, *National Public Radio.*

Cozolino, L. (2010). *The neuroscience of psychotherapy: Building and rebuilding the human brain.* New York, NY: W. W. Norton & Company.

Greshko, M., Parker, L., Howard, B. & Stone, D. (2018, August 2). A running list of how President Trump is changing environment policy. *National Geographic.*

Heintz, J. & Lewis, M. (2018, October 5). Nobel Peace Prize honors the fight against sexual violence. *America the Jesuit Review.*

Nianias, H. (2018, June 28). "Our men are leaving us": The Rohingya women facing life alone. *The Guardian.*

Prinz, W. (2012). *Open Minds: The Social Making of Agency and Intentionality.* Cambridge, MA: MIT Press.

Ricks, T. (2017). Looking back on my Navy career: From Tailhook scandal to Marines United. *Fp.*

Searcey, D. & Akinwotu, E. (2018, March 21). Boko Haram returns dozens of schoolgirls kidnapped in Nigeria. *The New York Times.*

Sher, J. (2013). *Somebody's daughter: The hidden story of America's prostituted children and the battle to save them.* Chicago, IL: Chicago Review Press.

Thompson, C. M. (2003). *Psychoanalysis: Evolution and development, with a new introduction by Paul Roazen.* New Brunswick, NJ and London: Transaction Publishers.

Van Natta, D. Jr. (1992, August 24) (rewritten August 17, 2017). *Miami Herald.*

EPILOGUE

A new collaboration

On my trip to the South I learned a great deal about past and present moment experiences as well as the importance of looking ahead. With regard to all three elements of time, I thought of another idea that had been interesting to me since I read Freud's *Project for a Scientific Psychology* (often referred to simply as *The Project*) when I was in analytic training more than 30 years ago and the new ways that neuroscience and psychoanalysis are coming together again in the form of neuropsychoanalysis, a union Freud struggled with off and on for much of his life. Solms, an internationally renowned psychoanalyst and neuroscientist, who trained initially as a scientist and more or less stumbled upon *The Project* (which led to his interest and training in psychoanalysis), believes this is the time to continue the discussion between these two fields. He has done this in New York by leading a neuropsychoanalysis discussion group which he started in 2001 (Schwartz, 2015).

In terms of the new relationship, sometimes the neuroscientists and psychoanalysts are even joined by attachment and listening-theory experts. Attention to mentalization has also arisen from the use (among other tools) of brain-imaging techniques like fMRI—functional magnetic resonance imaging—to measure activity in different areas of the working brain.

As research methodologies and instruments are further refined, it is likely that neurosciences will shed new light on the function of mentalization in human relationships, beyond the role of communication, which is Spunt's particular interest (2013). His preliminary findings already have strong implications for understanding how mentalization can function in the therapeutic dyad, as well as in intimate and personal relationships that require deep acceptance of the humanity of the other.

With regard to the renewed relationship I have mentioned, there also appears to be a great deal of potential in the "taking back of projections." Louis

Cozolino (2010) most succinctly highlights the essence of what is relevant about this topic.

> In therapy we teach our clients to ask themselves if the pot is calling the kettle black; that is, are their thoughts and feelings about others autobiographical? While in couples therapy we encourage our clients to stop mindreading to actually ask their partners what is on their minds. We created a parallel process whenever we explore how much of our reaction to a client is countertransferential. In our training as therapists, we learn to question our judgment and assumptions in light of our own personal histories. We also learn to use mirror neurons and theory of mind to enhance our attunement with our clients and explore their inner worlds; taking back our projections and working with transference and countertransference in therapy allows us to use our thoughts about others as potential sources of personal information.
>
> *(Cozolino, 2010, p. 315)*

In new connections we make with others, perhaps my idea of experience is also part of the union between neuroscience and psychoanalysis, since it too appears to include elements of brain functioning. Cozolino describes how Le Deux's theory of interpersonal relationships applies:

> As the core of our social brains, the amygdala organizes the appraisal of what we have learned from our relationship history. In interpersonal situations, our amygdala reflectively and unconsciously appraises others in the context of our past experiences. From moment to moment, the reflexive activations of our fast system (organized by past learning) shape the nature of our present experiences (Bar et al., 2006). This is a powerful mechanism by which our early social learning influences our experiences of the present.
>
> *(Cozolino, 2010, p. 244)*

The coming together of neuroscience and psychoanalysis makes perfect sense since Freud never meant for the separation to be permanent (Solms, 2015). He anticipated that one day advances in science would make it possible for his original hypotheses to be realized (Solms, 2015).

As stressful as the world is on various fronts, these are exciting times from a neuropsychoanalytic perspective. To live in a world where it could be commonplace to know that one's thoughts are not the thoughts of others would be truly remarkable. Such possibility would offer hope for so many who are mired in all types of projective processes, not yet close to knowing about the benefits of mentalizing and how such a capacity could be life-altering.

References

Cozolino, L. (2010). *The neuroscience of psychotherapy: Building and rebuilding the human brain.* New York, NY: W. W. Norton & Company.
Schwartz, C. (2015, August 25). When Freud Meets fMRI. *The Atlantic.*
Solms, M. (2015). *The feeling brain.* London and New York, NY: Routledge Press.
Spunt, R. P. (2013). Mirroring, mentalizing, and the social neuroscience of listening. *International Journal of Listening, 27,* 61–72.

INDEX

abandonment, fear of 16
abuse 25–28, 30–31, 50–52, 71, 72, 99–107, 112–113
action replacing thought 12
aggression: children learning to handle 119; and colonialism 100; and Donald Trump 69; genocide in Rwanda 99–107; groups 94, 95; and mentalization 117, 118, 119–120, 138; Northbrook Academy 97; and projective identification 11, 12, 13, 16, 19; repair of groups 122; and terrorism 124
Ainsworth, Mary 111
air force, women in 87–93, 155–156
Akerlof, Professor 55
Alford, C. Fred 13, 113, 122, 123, 124, 125, 135
Allen, Jon 3, 4, 116, 117, 118, 119, 134, 138
alpha process 20, 118
American Economic Association 62
American Psychiatric Association 34, 74
American Psychoanalytic Association 71
amygdala 163
anger 16, 105, 119, 120
Annan, Kofi 100
annihilation 11
anxiety 12, 73, 124, 133, 140
applied mentalization 134
Armenian genocide 127
Arnold, Henry H. 87, 89, 90, 91
Aron, Lewis 23, 26, 33, 37, 39, 154

attachment: attachment circuitry 4; attachment trauma 112–113; and epistemic trust 1; and mentalization 115–116, 118–119, 124, 137–152; secure attachment 111–112, 113–115; in therapeutic setting 3, 131–136, 155
Atwood, Margaret 7, 98
Aveling, Edward 47–48, 50–52

Backpage 105
badness within 11, 18, 100, 106, 112, 159
Balint, Michael 27, 29–30, 36
Balkan Wars 101
Barone, Michael 67
Basic Position 17
basic urges 137
Baun, Aleta 126
Beard, J. 48
Becker, Marie 80
Berry, Raymond H. 82
bias 2, 54, 56–57, 60, 61, 62
Biden, Joe 66
Bion, Wilfred 13, 20, 100, 118
bizarre objects 100
Black Lives Matter 66
blame 33, 71, 72, 82, 83, 105
Blow, Charles M. 65
blue-collar/working classes 48–49, 66, 67, 71, 80, 83, 155
Bohleber, Werner 112, 113, 132
Boko Haram 156
Bolz, Edna 80
Bowlby, John 111, 139

Brabant, E. 35, 37
Brandeis, Louis 67
Brazile, Donna 67–68
Brennan, B. William 25, 27, 29, 30, 32–33, 34–35, 36–38, 39
Budapest 22, 25
Byers, Eben 81

Camille 145–150
capitalism 47, 49, 155
Case, Anne 2, 53–63
Chernyshevsky, Nikolai 49
child development 13, 16, 94, 111, 118–119, 138–139; *see also* attachment
child labor 49–50
child sexual abuse 25–28, 30–31, 105
Chodorow, Nancy 38
Christie, Chris 70
civil society 71
Clark, C. 79
Clinton, Bill 66
Clinton, Hillary 64–75, 155
CNN 68, 92
Cochran, Jackie 87, 88
co-creation of stories 132
Cohen, Abby Joseph 57
Cold War 84
Collins, Eileen 91
collusion 97
Colombia 125
colonialism 100
Coman, Katharine 56
Comey, James 65, 68, 73
comfort women 102
Committee on the Status of Women in the Economics Profession (CSWEP) 56, 63
communication breakdown 13
compassion 39, 138
Constitution, US 64
Consumers League 82
containment 20, 118
Conti-Brown, Peter 55
control of others 7, 14, 154, 159
coping strategies 133, 134–135
corruption 65, 67
countertransference 14, 31, 35, 41, 154, 163
Cozolino, Louis 4, 132, 135, 159, 162–163
cultural, knowledge is 1, 2, 60, 131–132
cultural identities 99
cultural phenomenon, PTSD as 123–124
cultural traditions 95
Curie, Marie 60
Currie, Janet 62

Dallaire, Roméo 99, 100, 101, 125
Damasio, A. 4
Davenport, A. 137
Davidson, Adam 54
death of the psyche 112
Deaton, Angus 2, 53, 58–59
decoupling 112
defenses 15, 132, 137
dehumanization 101, 102
democracy 50, 52, 65
demonization 123–124, 125
Demuth, Freddy 51
denial 106, 127
depressive position 12, 16, 19, 94, 116, 117, 120
derivative processes 14
desensitization 131, 132
Deutsch, Helene 24
dial painters 79–86, 155
Dickens, Charles 26
DiNicola, Jennifer 106
discrimination 68, 97, 98
distancing 96–97
distorted thinking 12, 18, 95
Donohue, Catherine 82
Drinker, Cecil 80–81
Drinker, Katherine 81
drumming 126
Dukeshire, Theodore 24
Dupont, J. 25, 27, 28, 29, 32, 35

Earhart, Amelia 87
economics, women in 53–63
education of women 48, 50, 55–58
ego 137
Einstein, Albert 13
Electoral College 64–65
emancipation of women 49
emotional abuse 71, 72, 112
emotional regulation skills 133
emotional suffering 105–107
empathy 15, 39, 84, 116, 138
enactment 26, 33
enemies 13, 73, 101, 102, 123
Engels, Friedrich 45, 46, 47, 49, 51
envy 24
epistemic trust 1
equality 48, 49, 53, 62, 156
ethical codes 34
ethnic cleansing 156–157
ethnic hatred 94
evidence-based practice 26, 27, 131, 134
existential crisis 18
expendability of women 83

experience, learning from 12, 19, 118, 131, 143, 160
exposure techniques 131

fake news 65
false information 26, 65
family relationships 16–17
fantasy 14, 27, 74, 97, 116, 120, 154, 157, 158, 159
fathers: and attachment 114; father figures 26; Grayson and Camille 145–150; Trump's 73
feelings, acknowledging 114–115
female sexuality 24, 34, 106
femininity, in economics 61
feminism 24, 45, 68–69, 156
Ferenczi, Sándor 22–23, 25, 26–28, 31–37, 39, 116, 119, 154
Filipovic, Jill 71
Flinn, Franklin 81
fluctuating mental states 94
Fonagy, Peter 1, 3, 4, 112, 116, 117, 118, 138
Ford, Christine Blasey 160
foremothers, disparaging 30
foremothers, honoring 24, 68–69
forgiveness 125
Fort, Cornelia 88
Founders, US 64
Fox News 71
fragmentation 12, 112
Frankfurt School 122
"free love" 50
"free thinkers" 47
Freud, Anna 36
Freud, Sigmund 21, 22, 23, 28, 29, 31, 35, 36, 37, 39, 123, 137, 162, 163
Fromm, Erich 21, 22
Fromm-Reichmann, Freida 21
Fryer, Grace 81–82
fusion 116

Gabbard, G. 30, 31, 32
Gandhi, Mahatma 123
ganging up 7
gaslighting 155
Gelles, R. 26
Gelman, Andrew 53
gender discrimination 68–69, 98
genocide 99–107, 124–128, 156–157
German, A. B. 49
Gillibrand, Kirsten 73
Goldin, Claudia 54, 58, 62
Gornick, V. 46, 50–51

gossip and hearsay 26, 34
Gourevitch, Philip 101
grandiosity 19, 73, 74
Grayson and Camille 145–150
grief 120, 125
Grier, David Alan 91
Grossman, Leonard 82
Grotstein, J. 14
guilt 28, 52, 83, 96, 97, 105, 140

Hamilton, Alice 82
Han, Byung-Chul xi
Handmaid's Tale, The (Atwood, 1985) 7, 98
Hanrahan, Marion 88
hard truths, admitting to 125
Harmon, Elaine 88, 91
Harmon, Terry 91
Harris, A. 26, 33, 37, 39
Hartmann, Heidi 57
Haynal, André 39–40
healing groups 94–98
Hengel, Erin 62
Holmes, Rachel 45, 46, 47, 48, 49, 50, 51
hope 118, 122–128, 139
Horney, Karen 24
Hoxby, Caroline 58
Hugo, Pieter 103
human trafficking 103–104, 156
hurricanes 157–158

id 137
idealization 17
identity, cultural 99
ideology 95
immigrants 80
immobilization 124
industrial accidents 82, 83, 84
industrial revolution 48–49
Ingoma Nishya 126
inner other 113, 135, 155
Institute for Women's Policy and Research 57
intention 119, 135, 159
Interahamwe 100–101
internationalism 47
interpersonal psychoanalysis 21, 23, 116, 163
intersubjective moments 131
introjection 14
Inzozi Nziza 126
ISIS 156

Janie 139–141
Joanie 104–105

journalism 54, 58, 61, 67, 91, 155, 157

Kagame, Paul 125
Kapp, Y. 46, 47, 48, 51
Katese, Odile 126
Katz, Lawrence 54
Kavanaugh, Brett 160
Kernberg, Otto 14
King, Colbert I. 104
King, Martin Luther 123
"Kissing Technique" 29, 32, 34
Klein, Melanie 12–13, 14, 16, 19, 94–95, 117, 118, 122, 123, 124, 133
Kreps, Juanita 57
Kristof, Nicholas 105

La Porte, Irene 84
labor movements 47
Lady and the Unicorn, The 137
Landdeck, K. S. 91
Larice, Albina 80
Laurvik, Elma 31, 33, 36
leadership, women in positions of 38, 50, 155, 156
leaky pipeline effect 56
Lenin, Vladimir Ilych 49
LGBTQ 7, 66
Lippmann, Walter 82
listening, theory of 4, 119
London National Society for Women's Suffrage 48
Looney, Peg 80, 81, 84
Lowell, Alice 41n4
Lynch, Loretta 65

Madden, K. K. 56–57
Maggia, Amelia 80, 81, 84
magical thinking 134
Mandela, Nelson 123, 125
Martland, Harrison 82
Marx, Eleanor 45–52, 80, 154, 155
Marx, Karl 45, 46, 47, 49, 51
McHugh, John 91
media 67, 83–84, 85, 90, 91, 103, 123, 156
Meltzer, Donald 13
mentalization: and attachment 115–116, 118–119, 124, 137–152; and "back projections" 52; conditions for 138–139; and Donald Trump 161; as foundation for thinking 116–118; groups 95–98, 122, 123, 124–128; and the inner other 113; interpreting people's past actions 33–34; and non-mentalizing 119–120;

Shapiro on Thompson 25; in the therapeutic dyad 119; in therapeutic setting 3–4, 117, 131–136, 154–155
Messina, K. 2, 23
metacognition 135
metaphor 131, 138
Meyer, Adolf 34
Meyers Treatment Center 153
military women 87–93, 155–156
Mill, John Stuart 48
mirroring 111, 131, 132
Mitchell, Stephen 22, 37
Monica and Charles 141–145
Moore, Kate 79, 80, 81, 82, 83, 84, 85
Moss, Donald 71
mothers: and attachment 111–112, 114; Ferenczi's 32, 33; Thompson's 35; Trump's 73
Moulton, Ruth 23–24
mourning 12, 19, 118, 120, 140
Mundy, L. 61–62

Nader, Ralph 54
nannies 142, 144
narratives 132, 135, 159
National Runaway Switchboard (NRS) 106
neo-Freudians 154
neuroscience 4, 119, 132, 162
neurosis 15
New York Times 54, 62, 65, 68, 71, 104, 105
Newton's Laws of Thermodynamics 13
Nobel Prizes 54, 58–59, 60–63, 125, 160
nonjudgmental environment 4
non-mentalizing 119–120
non-verbal communication 119
Northbrook Academy 95–99
notes, publication of analysts' private 27, 35
not-me 11, 119
nuclear weapons 73, 84

Obama, Barack 55, 104, 156
Oedipal complex 28
Ogden, T. H. 14
one-body situation 14–15, 18, 19
one-mind, two minds process 52, 134, 143, 145
Ostrom, Elinor 61
other: destruction of the 19, 95, 101, 102; identification with 118; perceived "badness" of 123; as a whole person 17, 117, 120, 133

other side of the eye 157–158
outsiders, women economists as 57

Pálos, Gizella 33, 35–36
paranoid-schizoid position 12, 16, 19, 94, 95, 116, 117, 120
participant-observer relationship 23
patience 114, 119, 138
patient notes 27–28, 29, 31
patriarchy 2, 64
Pavia, W. 73
Paxson, Christina 59
Payne, Pearl 80
penis envy 24
Perkins, Frances 82
persecution, fear of 12
personality destruction 112
Petrova, Daniela 105
PhDs earned by women 56
Phillip, Adam 30
philosophy 117
physical abuse 99–107
pilots, female 87–93, 155–156
pleasure principle 123
Plotz, David 54
positions, Kleinian 12, 16, 94, 116, 117
post-traumatic stress disorder 123–124, 133
present-moment experience 131, 138
primitive processes 12, 14, 18
Prinz, Wolfgang 111, 159
projection 14, 15
projective identification: and Clara Thompson 34, 39; described 11–20; dial painters 83; and Eleanor Marx 50–52; genocide 100, 106; and Hillary Clinton 65, 72–73; Northbrook Academy 95–98; and women economists 61
property ownership 48, 106, 147
prostitution 49, 102, 103–105, 156
protective denial 106
psychological abuse 71
psychosis 15
Purcell, Charlotte Nevins 80

racism 71, 94, 96–98, 99, 100
radium girls 79–86, 155
rape 101–107, 156–157
rational thinking 19, 118, 120
Rawlinson, Mabel 88
reclamation of feelings 12
reconciliation 103, 124–127, 157
redactional identification 135–136, 159
reflection 132
regret 122

relational psychoanalysis 23, 31, 116
relationships: and attachment trauma 112; and Kleinian positions 13; and mentalization 116–118, 119; with one's self 138; participant-observer relationship 23; and projective identification 14–15, 155; therapist-patient 3, 21, 33, 119, 163
remorse 122
repair 3, 12, 19, 94–98, 118, 120, 122–128
reparative leadership 122–128, 157
repression of memory 26
reverse swarming 98
Ride, Sally 91
ridicule 25
Rivlin, Alice 57
Roazen, Paul 36, 41, 153, 154
Robinson, Joan 56
Roeder, Arthur 81, 82, 83
role models 58, 97
Romer, Christina D. 57
Romero, J. 55–56
Russian electoral interference, alleged 65
Rwanda 99–107, 124–127, 156–157

Santos, Juan Manuel 125
Sawhill, Isabel 57
scapegoating 97
Schaub, Katherine 80
second-wave feminism 4–5, 53
self-awareness 113, 115–116, 133, 138, 156, 157
self-erasure 12
self-esteem 19, 73
self-other boundary 15
self-reflection 138
self-worth 106
senators 62
sexism 62, 67
sex-trafficking 103–107, 156
sexual abuse 25–28, 30–31, 105
sexual contact therapist-patient 25, 28, 29, 30, 32, 33, 35–37
sexual harrassment 62, 71, 98, 160
shame 72, 105–106, 115
Shapiro, Susan 25–26, 27, 29–31, 32, 34, 35, 38, 39
Shatterly, Margot Lee 91
Sher, J. 106, 107, 156
Shults, Tammie Jo 92
slavery 64, 104
social brains 163
social justice 47
social media 7, 68, 73, 74
social mirroring 111

socialism 47, 49, 50, 52, 154
Solms, M. 162, 163
South Sudan 103
splitting 14
Spunt, R. P. 4, 119, 162
Sri Lanka 123
Steele, B. F. 113
Steinem, Gloria 74
STEM 62–63, 91
stereotypes 2, 57
Stevenson, Betsey 62
storytelling 131–132, 135, 159
Strickland, Donna 160
subjective experience 1–2, 4, 143
suffrage 48, 49, 50, 64
suicide 50, 51, 52
Sullenberger, Sully 92
Sullivan, Harry Stack 21, 22–23, 116, 119
Sunni-Shia conflict 126–127
superego 113
Supreme Court 160
"swarming" 98

taking back: and mentalization 98, 117, 118, 119, 120, 160, 161, 162–163; and projective identification 12, 14, 19; reconciliation 125
Taylor, Eugene 23, 26, 32, 35
terrorism 123–124
Thaden, Louise 87
therapeutic alliance 3, 155
Thomas, G. 73
Thompson, Clara 21–41, 116, 119, 153–154, 155
Thorne, Will 47
thriving 138
trade unions 47, 50
transference 14, 15, 153, 163
trauma: attachment trauma 112–113; exposure techniques 131; Ferenczi's concepts of 27; and immobilization 124; long-term effects of 26; and mentalization 131–136; post-traumatic stress disorder 123, 133
Trump, Donald: attitudes to women 69–72, 98, 160–161; grandiosity 19, 73, 74; and Hillary Clinton 64, 67–68, 70, 72–73; and Janet Yellen 55; mentalizing 161; and projective identification 18–20; Russian electoral interference, alleged 65; and terrorism 124; and workplace harm 155
trust 65, 66, 138
Twitter 68, 73, 74

two-body processes 14–15, 16, 18, 19
two-person psychology 21, 116, 119
Tyson, Laura D'Andrea 57

umuganda 125
unconditional love, children need 138
unconscious, the 2, 14, 18, 72
unconscious bias 2, 54, 60
unions 47, 50
universal suffrage 48, 50
unpublished work 38–39
Ursano, Bob 153
US Constitution 64
US Founders 64
US Senate 61–62
Uvin, Peter 100–101

Van Dam, A. 55
Van Natta Jr, Don 157–158
van Neumann Whitman, Martina 57
verbal violence 71–72
victim-blaming 38
Victoria, Queen 48
violence: and aggressive feelings 13; as a concept xiii ; at the hands of men 14; healing groups 94; and projective identification 13; verbal violence 71–72; *see also* aggression
voting rights 48, 64

wartime rape 101–102
Washington School of Psychiatry (WSP) 21, 24, 38, 153
weaving occupation 126
Weinstein, Harvey 71
Weiss, Edoardo 12
West Timor 126
whole person 17, 117, 120, 133
"wife," use of 54
Wiley, Katherine 82
William Alanson White Institute 24, 38
Wilson, Michael 104
Wolfers, Justin 54–55
Wollstonecraft, Mary 48
women: Eleanor Marx and the "woman question" 48; and Nobel Prizes 60–61; psychological differences from men 23–24; senators 62
women pilots 87–93, 155–156
Women's Air Service Pilots (WASP) 87–93, 155–156
women's cooperatives 126
Women's March Washington 74

Women's Movement 69
women's rights 48, 49–50, 64, 106
working classes 48–49, 66, 67, 71, 80, 83, 155
World War I 102
World War II 87–93, 102
Wu, Alice 62

Yellen, Janet 54–55, 59, 61, 62
Yousafzai, Malala 160
Yulín Cruz, Carmen 73

Zhang, Sarah 83
Ziba 102–103
Zinner, John 14, 15, 18, 73

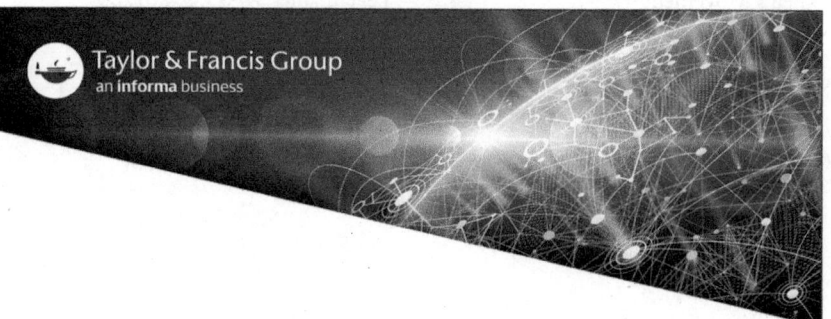